YOUR SECOND LIFE

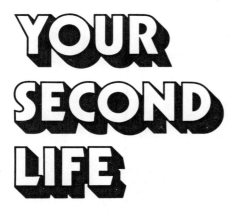

YOUR SECOND LIFE

Harold L. Karpman, M.D.
and Sam Locke

PUBLISHED BY J. P. TARCHER, INC., LOS ANGELES

Distributed by Hawthorn Books, Inc., New York

Dedications:
To my lovely family--may their creative efforts,
individually and collectively, surpass this one . . .
and to my patients, for their inspiration and trust.

−H.L.K.

To my mother, Mrs. Jennie Locke.

−S.L.

Acknowledgments:
To Mrs. Jean McNeil, my secretary at the inception of the
project; my current secretary, Ms. Nanci Wright, for all her
superb help; and, last but not least, to my stenographer,
Ms. Marge "Flying Fingers" Belanger.

−H.L.K.

To Esther-Jane Lustig for her research and constructive
criticism.

−S.L.

Contents

1. Your Second Life

Long ago, when I was in residency training in a Boston hospital, an eminent local physician, a Harvard cardiologist, loved to regale us with stories of one of his patients.

"Whenever I came into his ward," he said, "he was always devouring the same book. The minute he'd see me, he'd pop the book under his pillow before I had a chance to see the title. Naturally I was curious, and one day I said, 'Come on, Mario. I'm over twenty-one. At least let me look at the pictures.' He sheepishly took the book out. It wasn't pornographic at all. It was a cardiology text for medical students." The cardiologist laughed. "The son of a gun was checking up on my treatment to make sure I was doing the right things for him."

I have been reminded of this story with increasing frequency over the last few years whenever I've seen a patient with his nose buried in a cardiac text, a text generally written for the lay reader. But no one has bothered to slide the book under the pillow when I approach. If anything, the patient, or frequently members of the family, have asked me to *clarify* some points they thought vague or confusing.

But physicians are slowly beginning to realize that patients are actually like members of a minority group and that their interest in the physiology and pathology of their ailments, their refusal to accept uncritically the Medical Word From On High, indicates that, like members of other minorities, they want more say in the decisions affecting their lives.

Patients *need* to be better informed about their condition—not so that they can practice medicine, but so they can actively participate with their physicians in leading them out of, or preventing them from entering, the sticky morass of ill health. A physician is practicing good medicine when he actively informs and educates his patients.

The practice of medicine today is, because of its very sophisticated nature, outside the everyday experience of most people. It has become for them supersaturated with an increasing amount of mystery and "abracadabra." Not enough doctors, I feel, make an effort to simplify, to explain to their patients what is happening to them and, equally important, what is being done for them. Indeed, some doctors do not see the need for it or assign it its proper importance.

Unfortunately every ointment invariably has a fly. Though I have vigorously encouraged patients to read popular books about their disorders, I have discovered that few read much beyond the first thirty pages before putting them down for good. Why? Because the books provide more information than patients can absorb, often require more concentration than they can maintain (especially if they're in a convalescing state), and, last but not least, they are frequently terribly boring. Patients find these books difficult to read even though they are intended for laymen because they are, for all of these reasons, *doctor* oriented. They are written to educate, but usually presented in a formal, pedantic, "doctor-like" fashion.

I decided therefore that it was time for a book that is *patient* oriented. Sometimes it is hard to realize that the focal point of the health care system, the vast medical apparatus assembled during this final quarter of the century, *is* the patient. As specialists and superspecialists have multiplied, the depersonalization of the doctor-patient relationship has increased. One surgeon told me how a handsome woman came up to him at a party and reminded him that he had performed an operation on her knee cap only a few months earlier. To his embarrassment he could not remember her. He could recall the diagnosis, the instruments, the area he'd operated on, but not the face.

Fifty years ago humorist Irvin Cobb, in his hilarious "Speaking of Operation," described the patient's view of specialists thus:

> . . . up-to-date practitioners just go ahead and divide you up and partition you out among themselves without saying anything to you about it. Your torso belongs to one man and your legs are the exclusive property of his brother practitioner down on the next block, and so on. You may belong to as many as half a dozen specialists, most of whom, very possibly, are total strangers to you, and yet never know a thing about it yourself.
>
> It has rather the air of trespass—nay, more than that, it bears some of the aspects of unlawful entry—but I

suppose it is legal. Certainly judging by what I am able to learn, the system is being carried on generally. So it must be ethical.

It *is* ethical, but it is certainly not as personal and doctors are becoming more aware that they must deal not only with the part affected but with the person affected as well. As one surgeon put it, "We don't operate on hearts, we operate on people."

Unfortunately, because of the need for more specialists, re-personalizing doctor-patient relationships has become more difficult. Doctors just don't have time. The old wheeze about the doctor telling a patient he must have long periods of rest and the patient answering, "I'll get it in your waiting room," isn't funny anymore. It's getting to be too true. As much as I believe in the importance of explaining treatment to patients, I know that when I'm doing it in depth with one patient I am taking time from another. And I know that when I'm not doing it adequately, I'm practicing less than one-hundred percent medicine.

This book, then, is an attempt to give patients the time they deserve—and to do it in a way that, I hope, you will find entertaining as well as instructive. Realizing that the pace of living has quickened and that the reading attention-span of many of us has lessened (yes, for doctors as much as patients), my collaborator, Sam Locke, and I have tried to convey medical knowledge by presenting it as a series of dramatic dialogues. For the most part these dialogues, which are based on actual cases, have purposefully been limited to the most prevalent forms of cardiac disorders—those that would apply to most readers of this book. They are presented pretty much as they actually happened, although we have simplified them, modified the dialogue, sometimes changed the time sequences, and the like, in order to best illuminate the problems of the heart and the heart patient.

Through dialogue and action, we have tried to delineate the major behavior areas and lifestyles that seem frequently to be associated with heart problems. I have woven into the text the questions heart-attack victims often ask me and the answers I usually give them. I have reviewed factors in patients' ailments which they think are beyond their control but which are not. I have tried to convey how much patients can do for themselves, how important their actions are in their recovery, and how the value of an appropriately close collaboration with their doctor can extend into the post-coronary life. A glossary gives the most common cardiac terms, and appendices present frequent questions heart patients ask about sex, diet, exercise, and smoking.

What is important to remember is that the life after the heart attack, the second life as it were, is not second best, second class, or second rate. If anything, it can be *better* than the first. Often, patients return long after their recovery and tell me that if it hadn't been for their heart attack, they would never have had the incentive to restructure their relationships and habits, to develop a life after their heart attack which was much more satisfying and meaningful than what had existed before their coronary. Their heart attack proved to be the stimulus they needed to throw off the shackles of a confining and pressureful life.

If critical areas are left intact, we probably could get along quite well even with severely damaged hearts, operating with perhaps no more than twenty-five percent of the heart muscle remaining uninjured. More often than not, the capacity of the wounded heart is less critical in achieving a good second life than is the capacity of the mind to bring understanding, faith, and resolution to the challenge. A twenty-five percent heart can frequently make it with a one-hundred percent attitude.

Finally, we hope this book will help prevent some non-patients from becoming patients. If reading about people with disastrous life habits can inspire a change sufficient to ward off a coronary crisis, that is justification enough for this book.

2. A Bolt from the Blue

It started, as it frequently does, with a buzz from my secretary on the intercom.

"Mr. Justin is on the phone, Doctor. He's complaining of chest discomfort."

Frank Justin, forty-four years old. I'd met him at the tennis club several times. He was a plump man, but thickly built rather than flabby. He was a dress manufacturer, an executive in soft goods, but there was nothing soft about him. Even his tennis game was driving: 6-0 was his favorite score. He was known for a sardonic sense of humor, although at the moment it was not evident.

"Hi, Harold, I know you're probably busy, but I just wanted to check something with you quick. I've been feeling kinda lousy these last couple days, had a lot of indigestion, and I just wondered . . ."

"Indigestion? After every meal?"

"What? No, mostly after lunch."

"But not after dinner?"

"Ah, actually, I haven't been eating much dinner for the past two or three days."

"Why not?"

"Too bushed by the time I get home."

"How long has this been going on?"

"I told you. Two or three days, maybe longer." His voice became hesitant. "Matter of fact, I've been feeling kinda bad all week."

"I see." I shifted the phone to pick up a pencil. "What about the chest pains my secretary said you mentioned? How long have you had them?"

"About two days. And I didn't tell her 'pains'; I said 'discomfort,' although it did become kind of a pain today."

"When today?"

"About half an hour ago. I was coming back from lunch, crossing the street. The lights changed and I had to run for the curb and I got this pain in my chest."

"Is it still there?"

"Sort of. I took an Alka-Seltzer and a Tums. I even took some aspirin. Look, I didn't want to bother you with this, but this crazy secretary of mine dialed your number and just handed me the phone. I didn't want to waste your time. As a matter of fact I hope I *am* wasting your time . . ."

Frank isn't the first executive who's told of his secretary phoning the doctor and then handing him the phone before he could cancel the call. Either there are a lot of aggressively solicitous secretaries or most businessmen are too reluctant to admit self-concern. Why do so many patients believe the doctor is wasting his time listening to symptoms when that's his job—when the symptoms may indicate that a life is in danger? When Frank told me he didn't want to bother me, it wasn't just me he was reluctant to disturb, it was himself, too. He simply didn't want to admit there might be something the matter with him.

"Where is the pain right now, Frank?"

"In the chest, like I said, though right now it's a lot less than before. Maybe it's nothing."

"Where exactly in the chest?"

"The lower part, in the middle, just above the belly. But it's hardly even a pain any more."

"Then what is it?"

"More like something was pressing on my chest. Maybe it'll go away."

I had written on my desk pad, *Frank Justin. Acute myocardial infarction?*—which is the medical name for heart attack. I also wrote the name of the hospital closest to Frank's business.

"Does this pain or feeling go anywhere else?"

"Well, it sort of spreads up to my shoulders and neck."

"Is that all?"

"Well, not exactly."

"What do you mean 'not exactly'?"

"Well, sometimes it shoots down to my left elbow. But mainly it presses on my chest, though it doesn't hurt like it did."

Each person perceives physical discomfort in his own way, of course. Some, like Frank, feel a heart attack as pressure on the chest. Others feel as if their insides are being squeezed or as if they have stabbing pains in the stomach or in the back muscles. Occasionally there may be nausea or vomiting, sometimes even the feeling that the heart is on fire.

My initial impression was that Frank was in the early

stages of a heart attack, but it was still possible that he was only suffering from indigestion, gall bladder trouble, or some other benign, less threatening disorder.

"Frank, have you had anything like this happen to you at any time during this past year or so?"

"Well, last winter when Sheila and I were in Mexico City, the first day I got the same feeling. I figured it was the altitude. Half an hour it was gone."

"Was there any other time?"

"Jesus, Doc, are you doing my biography?"

"In a way." I shifted the phone again as I tore the page out of the pad. "Frank, chest symptoms like you have now, plus the pain in your shoulders and neck and left elbow, could be caused by several things, and once I get your medical history maybe I can figure which one. Now—was there any other time?"

"About two months ago I got it on the tennis court. It wasn't as bad as it was today, but it was bad. And another time when I was running for a cab. On my last trip to New York."

"If I remember from the club locker room, you're about, what—twenty-five pounds overweight?"

"Well, I don't know exactly," he said irritably, "but I'm active. At the office I'm on my feet a hell of a lot. Every weekend I play tennis. You've seen me, I mean I really play . . . you know, a lot of volleying . . ."

And now he was volleying with me.

I had enough history to make an educated guess. "Frank, I want you to get over to Memorial Hospital for a checkup."

"I don't know if I can fit it in this week—"

"I'm not talking about this week. I'm talking about right now."

" Right *now?*"

"My office is going to make the arrangements as soon as we get off the phone."

"Jesus, I haven't been in a hospital since I had my tonsils out. I mean, this is a real bolt from the blue."

"Get someone to take you over. I don't want you driving. When you get to the ambulance entrance, if there isn't a wheelchair waiting, have whoever is driving you go to the admitting office and get a wheelchair, and the attendant will take you right up to the Coronary Care Unit."

"Come on, Harold, what do I need a wheelchair for?"

"It's standard for a patient being admitted to the hospital to be wheeled to the examining room. You'll then change into a gown, and be given a cardiogram, x-rays, blood tests, temperature and blood pressure check, and some medication. It's all routine. I'll meet you there."

"You mean you want me to leave for the hospital right now?" I had a pretty good idea what to expect next and Frank didn't disappoint me. "Doctor, can I tell you what a load of work I've got to get off . . ."

"No, let me tell you. If you leave right now, the wheels stop turning, the firm goes bankrupt, and everybody's out on welfare."

"Jesus, all I ask is a couple of hours."

"Now, Frank."

"A half hour."

It's amazing how often the allegiance to work is stronger than the instinct for survival. But over fifty percent of the deaths caused by heart attacks occur in the first hours after they've begun, before the victim even reaches the hospital. And Frank seemed prepared to spend minutes of those precious hours arguing with me. I didn't tell him any of this, of course. More anxiety was nothing to lay on someone who might be having a heart attack even as I was talking to him.

"Frank," I said gravely, "I think you may be in the middle of a coronary spasm, and the sooner we start therapy the less chance of your developing complications."

"Coronary spasm" is one of those nonspecific medical terms that sobers people without panicking them. I added politely, "Would you like me to send an ambulance for you?"

"An ambulance! Hell, no! My wife'll drive me down. I'll phone her."

"No, get your partner, your secretary, or anyone at the office. Not your wife."

"Why not? She can be here in twenty minutes . . ."

"I don't want you waiting twenty minutes, Frank. Have your secretary call her to meet you at the hospital. And *get going,* will you!"

Later I learned that Frank had his accountant drive him, and, true to form, he had discussed business all the way.

When he arrived at the hospital, he was whisked in a wheelchair to the Coronary Care Unit and hooked to the EKG machine; the electrocardiogram could indicate to me if coronary damage had occurred or if the heart was malfunctioning in any way. Blood samples were also taken, along with his temperature and blood pressure. A needle was inserted in his forearm and an intravenous sugar solution was started.

By the time I arrived a few minutes later, his EKG was ready. It unequivocally revealed to me that he was suffering from an acute coronary—a heart attack, a myocardial infarction.

When I entered the CCU ward, Frank was in bed, with electrodes and tubes sprouting out of his body like weeds. Two EKG monitors, one at his bedside and one at the central nursing station, were beeping out his heart action and displaying constantly changing electrocardiograms on the oscilloscope screens.

Frank and I looked at each other, formerly casual acquaintances, now linked by a life and death situation.

"How'm I doin', Doc?" he mumbled. He had been given a mild sedative.

"Tell you in a minute, Frank."

The beeping EKG monitor told me his heart had stabilized satisfactorily. According to the nurse's notes, his temperature was normal, which is usual at that stage of a coronary. It doesn't start going up until twenty-four to forty-eight hours after a myocardial infarction, when the damaged heart commences repair activity. Then the temperature may climb to a level of three or four degrees above normal. Frank's breathing was normal; he wasn't panting or short of breath. He was pale, but there was no sign of cyanosis—lips and fingernails turning blue because of the heart being unable to pump enough blood through the body. I listened to his heart and lungs through the stethoscope, then examined his head, eyes, ears, nose, throat, abdomen, and extremities.

"I'd say your condition has stabilized," I said to Frank. "You're doing fine, under the circumstances."

"Under what circumstances?"

"Well, your lungs are clear, no fluid in them. Your hands and feet are O.K., no swelling. Your eyes are clear. Your blood pressure and temperature are normal though your temperature may go up. The point is, you're having a coronary, but judging from your condition it's only a small one."

"Doctor, in case you haven't heard, there's no such thing as a *small* coronary to a patient."

Frank was obviously less sedated than I had thought.

"O.K., let me explain. When I say you have a coronary, that's short for coronary thrombosis. A thrombosis is a blood clot that dams up the passageway of an artery from the heart. The tissue beyond the clog point, which that artery was supplying blood to, becomes injured because its supplies of oxygen and food are cut off. In your case, it looks like the amount of tissue affected is quite small, no larger than an almond. That's why I said I think you're having a small coronary."

"You *think* I'm having a small coronary." His emphasis left little doubt about what he thought of the state of my knowledge. The driving executive and tennis player in him were still in command, although he was beginning to look sleepy. Heart patients vary in their reactions; some panic, some are stoical, some are stunned, some philosophical, some deny they've had one altogether, and some react with anger. Frank was the last type.

"It'll take a few days before I can say I know for sure."

"And I have to stay here till then?"

I knew that at his age Frank must have been acquainted with enough people who had had coronaries to know that the first two or three days, at least, were spent in CCU. But his reflex was always to haggle for better terms.

"If you are having a coronary, Frank, and that's what it looks like to me, you'll probably be here anywhere from two days to a week. Then you'll go to a regular hospital room here and stay there about two or two and a half weeks. That's about how long it'll take your heart to heal."

"*That* long?"

"Frank," I asked, "did you ever lacerate an arm or a leg?"

"Boy, did I! I played ice hockey in high school, and I've

still got a scar on my ass where I was ripped by my own hockey stick. Would you like to see it?"

"Oh, I've seen lots of hockey sticks," I deadpanned. "How long did it take to heal?"

"Who remembers? About a month."

"Well, that's about the same amount of time it'll take your heart to heal. A heart attack is like a laceration. The attack damages an area of the heart muscle, and this heart muscle must heal and form a scar, just like the scar on your behind. It takes one to three weeks for that scar to form and become strong enough for the heart to carry on as usual. A fractured arm can be put in a cast and a lacerated buttock can be bandaged, but a heart can only be mended by reducing your activity. And no one yet has figured how to put the heart to bed for a rest without including the rest of the body."

"You mean I've got to treat my heart as good as I treated my ass."

"Right."

"Keep it in bed a month."

"Or whatever it takes."

"Why can't I go home to bed?"

It seems nobody loves home so much as when they're in a hospital.

"Look, Frank, you're in your early forties. You've still got close to half your life ahead of you. Think of this time in the hospital as an investment in that second lifetime. Complications can set in—especially in the first seventy-two hours."

"What kind of complications?"

"Frank, you're the first person I've seen trying to get a medical degree on his back. Now, if you'll promise to give that sedative a chance to work I'll answer this one last question."

"O.K., Doc, it's a deal."

"All right, at the onset of a heart attack, we're never absolutely sure if the heart has been weakened. Sometimes its rhythm can change or it gets too tired to keep up the circulation adequately. Well, in a hospital like this we're prepared to cope. We've got methods to help the heart's pumping temporarily, to correct any malfunction in its rhythm, and to carry it right through the critical period. We've also got the people who know how to use these devices. Once you've got past that critical period and you don't have to be watched every minute, you'll move to a regular hospital bed. When you're well enough, you'll sit up; then we'll get you up; and finally you'll be walking around, And *then* you get to go home. You know the adage, 'Today is the first day of the rest of your life'? Well, these three or four weeks here can be the *beginning* of a long healthy life."

Frank grinned up at me from the jungle of wires and tubes. "What you're trying to say is that it's a little harder to kick off in a hospital."

I smiled back. "No. What I'm saying is that it's a little easier to start a second life from here."

3. The Science of Guessing

I walked into the corridor outside the Coronary Care Unit and found Frank's wife, Sheila, a pretty, soft-faced woman approaching forty. With her were two of their children, Alex, sixteen, and Margot, twelve, plus a sharper-featured, better-groomed woman who was an older version of Sheila. There was also a small, white-haired woman of about seventy, with a stricken expression, who resembled Sheila. The fact that Sheila had such a large contingent with her could indicate either how close-knit the family was or how difficult it was for her to face a crisis alone, or both.

Whenever I step out of a hospital room to face a hastily summoned family, I try to counter the tension with a relaxed, reassuring manner. "Hello, Sheila," I said cheerfully. I had met her and the children at Frank's tennis club. "Everything's under control." I extended my hand to the old lady. "I'm Dr. Karpman. You must be Sheila's mother."

"Yes." She gave my hand a quick, anxious clutch.

"*Our* mother," the sharp-featured woman informed me. "I'm Sheila's sister, Lisa Mann."

"How do you do." I shook her hand and turned to Sheila. "Frank is doing all right now, from the looks of things. I think he's having what's called a myocardial infarction."

I have frequently found in the initial explanation of sudden heart ailments to a cardiac victim's family that technical terms like myocardial infarction are less upsetting than more common ones like heart attack, coronary thrombosis, or massive coronary.

"That's the same as coronary thrombosis, isn't it?" Lisa Mann asked. "I read that somewhere."

So much for the technical terminology approach.

"Well, yes, essentially. 'Myocardial' means heart muscle in Greek and 'infarction' is when the heart muscle is damaged by being deprived of blood."

"And that's what a coronary thrombosis means, doesn't it?"

"Pretty much," I said. "A thrombus is a blood clot. When it clogs up one of the heart arteries you get what's called coronary thrombosis, and that usually produces a myocardial infarction, a heart attack. Look, I know there are a lot of things you'll want to ask me. Why don't we go down to the lounge at the end of the floor and sit down?"

Sometimes I give the patient or the family more of an answer than they may expect. Usually they become less anxious if they know exactly what has happened and what might happen during the next forty-eight to seventy-two hours. Also, fuller explanations tend to distract people from their agitation and help calm them.

We sat down in the lounge and I spoke directly to Sheila.

"The plugging up of the artery means the tissue cells

beyond that stopped-up point are cut off from oxygen and food, like a river town left high and dry when the river is dammed above it. That damming up of an artery is called an occlusion; the artery is blocked."

Sheila watched me intently, but it was hard to tell how much she heard. Her lips, on which she'd forgotten to put lipstick, quivered slightly. I cut right to what would reassure her most quickly.

"Right now, Frank's resting comfortably. His condition has stabilized, his blood pressure is good, his temperature is as expected, there have been no complications . . ."

"Doctor, when will he be coming home?"

No questions about whether Frank was out of danger or still in pain, only "When will he be coming home?" Actually, it was a comparatively mild example of someone trying to avoid facing the shock of their spouse's condition. I've listened to wives' long discussions of which bathrobe and pajamas to bring back to their husbands in the hospital, to the effect of the heart attack on their vacation plans or even on the important dinner dance next Saturday night. But all are simply trying to dodge the reality of what has just happened.

"Sheila, if this turns out to be a heart attack, as I think it is, and if the healing process proceeds without complications, he should be home within two to three weeks."

"Three weeks." She let out a sigh. You could almost see the numbness beginning to melt. She turned to the others. "Three weeks." She turned back to me. "I hope you don't mind my bringing my family with me."

"I'm delighted. The more relatives show up to get it right from the horse's mouth, so to speak, the less chance details will get garbled when they're passed on to other members of the family. Also less chance of unasked questions you might think of later. Among the five of you there should be plenty of questions." I smiled encouragingly.

I never had an invitation accepted with more alacrity than Lisa Mann showed.

"Doctor," she said, "you keep saying things like '*if* this turns out to be a heart attack' . . . or you *think* he's having a coronary. Don't you know for sure?"

I shook my head. "Not yet."

"Well, when will you know?"

"Mrs. Mann, a person can have severe chest pain, palpitation, shortness of breath—that still doesn't prove it's a heart attack beyond the shadow of a doubt."

"Well, what does?"

"The electrocardiogram."

"What's that?" Twelve-year-old Margot had piped up. Her aunt gave her a slightly annoyed look.

"It's a strip of paper from a very important instrument," I said. "You see, the heart is run by electric power produced by millions of heart cells. That electricity is what controls the pumping of the chambers of the heart, what makes them expand and contract and push the blood around the body."

Marge nodded solemnly. "We studied the chambers of the heart in school."

"Good. Now, that electricity in the heart works in waves like . . ."

"Like one of those Christmas trees in the store window where the lights go around like in waves?" Margot suggested.

"Yes, very good, Margot. Excellent!" In spite of her worry about her father, the child glowed. "Now, when an electrocardiograph machine is attached to you, all the electric waves coming from all parts of your heart register on the strip of paper, the electrocardiogram. When anything happens to the heart, the electric waves change, the doctor can read the electrocardiogram, and from the way the waves are different on the chart he can tell just what is happening in the heart."

"Then why," asked Lisa, "can't you say for sure if Frank had a coronary or not?"

"Because when a heart suffers a coronary thrombosis, the effects on the electrical impulses of the heart is frequently not immediate. They may take up to three days to show up on the charts."

"Why so long?"

In terms of persistence, Lisa resembled her brother-in-law a lot more than she did her sister.

"It takes time for the change to develop," I said, "but when it does it's a foolproof way of ascertaining that a heart attack has occurred."

"Is that the only way?"

"No, there are other ways. The area of the heart that's damaged releases certain substances known as enzymes into the bloodstream. We can measure these enzymes and if they're abnormally elevated we know there's been a coronary. But sometimes other conditions can raise the blood levels of the enzymes, so we have to be careful in using that as the only way of diagnosing the heart attack. But, don't worry, we'll do all the tests."

Lisa sighed. "So right now you're not sure it's a coronary?"

"Not quite, but pretty sure. And we are treating him for it because all the symptoms point that way."

"But it could be something else?" Sheila said suddenly alert.

"It's not likely, but conceivably."

"Like what?"

"Well, maybe that coronary artery that we think is blocked isn't really blocked. It's still letting a little blood flow through. Not enough to keep the tissue healthy but enough to keep it from dying. That's called ischemia, or coronary insufficiency."

"Anything else?" Sheila asked, tense.

I shrugged. "It could be one or a combination of many other things. For example, a gall bladder attack, or ulcer, or attack of indigestion . . ."

"That's what it is!" Sheila interrupted. "Frank eats like a horse. You know how he eats, Mother."

Her mother nodded vigorously.

"He's a real fatty," Sheila said.

"Daddy isn't a fatty!" Margot countered shrilly.

"He's overweight, darling, and how many times have you heard me tell him to eat slower?" She turned to me. "It *is* indigestion."

"Not very likely," I said, but Sheila wasn't listening.

"If I've told him once, I've told him a thousand times, he's got to cut down, haven't I?" she appealed to her family. Her mother continued nodding her head. "No question that's what it is."

I wasn't sorry for Sheila's sudden euphoria, even if it was based on wishful thinking. It could carry her through the next few days until she became tough enough to handle the new realities. And her toughness, like that of all spouses of cardiac patients, would be vital.

Frank's gangling son, who had been staring at the floor most of the time, suddenly opened up. "Is my dad going to be all right, Doctor?" he said with a quaver.

I put a hand on his arm. "Let me put it this way, Alex.

I'd bet a dollar to a dime, he's going to come out all right. In an hour, I'd raise it to two dollars to a dime. By this time tomorrow, I'd make it twenty dollars. The day after tomorrow, if nothing happens, I'd make it fifty dollars."

"The odds get better all the time, huh?" He smiled.

"Doctor," said Lisa, "what do you mean 'if nothing happens'?"

The woman's antenna were never down.

"Well, so far Frank is doing well, but complications can occur in the early phases of a coronary. His heart could develop fast or irregular rhythms—arrhythmias they're called. Or the heart could lose some of its strength, its ability to pump the blood . . ."

"But, Doctor, you said the odds were getting better." Alex had lost his smile.

"They are. Every minute there's less chance of any of these things happening."

"But they could, couldn't they?"

"Yes. But that's why your dad's right here in CCU. All the nurses and doctors have been intensively trained in handling cardiac emergencies. The unit's equipped with oxygen and the latest drugs and machines, which are usually capable of handling complications. It's the best possible place for a man with a coronary to be, take my word for it."

"How could it be a coronary?" Sheila asked doggedly. "Frank's so healthy."

"He's too fat!" her sister said.

"Who said so?" Sheila asked indignantly.

"You did," Lisa replied. "Just a minute ago."

"What's that got to do with—with . . ."

"It's what brings on a coronary," Lisa declared. "You can read that in the papers every day."

"Jerry's fatter than Frank," Sheila retorted.

"But my husband doesn't push himself the way yours does!"

"Girls, girls, don't fight," the old lady said wearily. "It's not .. "

"Jerry says Frank is the hardest worker in the plant," Lisa went on. "Work, work, work. That's the type that gets heart attacks."

"Every weekend he plays tennis," Sheila came back. "Which is more than Jerry does."

"Frank pushes himself too hard," Lisa nodded smugly. "I tell Jerry, don't push yourself. I don't believe in pushing." It was an odd sentiment coming from such an aggressive woman. She suddenly turned to me. "Don't you think that pushing gives you coronaries, Doctor?"

"The exact reason why a person develops a heart attack is still uncertain," I said diplomatically. "Statistically we know it develops most frequently among people who have hypertension, diabetes, or a family history of heart disease— say a parent or grandparent who died of a heart condition or hypertension. We also know there are a lot of other factors statistically related to the development of heart trouble."

"Pushing is one of them, right?" Lisa inquired eagerly.

"There's no question stress can contribute to a coronary. So can overwork, especially if the work is aggravating and unpleasant to you. So can an inability to relax, a too-powerful drive for success." Lisa gave her sister a smirk. "On the other hand so can overweight, a sedentary life, too much cholesterol in the blood, cigarette smoking. Each of these factors has been associated with heart trouble. Often a few of them can be found in each case and the importance of each varies. A fat man who smokes a pack a day and works ten hours a day has a heart attack. Which factor caused it? Any one of them, but probably all of them together. We can't tell. There are nearly 700,000 cases of myocardial infarction in this country a year, and no two of them are exactly alike because the importance of these factors vary from person to person."

"Why hasn't the medical profession invented something that can analyze the factors in each case?" Lisa asked indignantly.

"They have," I told her. "The cardiologist. We're the invention that does it. We add up the symptoms plus the nature of the patient, his qualities, his attitudes toward his work, his family, his friends, his family history, whether or not he smokes, many things. We run that through our training and experience, exercise our judgment, our intuition as it were, and come up with an impression. The cardiogram and blood tests usually tell us whether that impression is correct."

"Sounds to me like guesswork," sniffed Lisa.

"You're right," I said. "It's like what it says on an old medical school diploma. It was given for studying not the science of medicine but the *art* of medicine. Art is judgment, intuition, educated guesswork. And within three days, maybe even by tomorrow, we'll know if my educated guess about Frank is right."

Lisa turned to Sheila. "Are you going to let his family know?" She looked at me. "He's got two brothers in New York," she explained.

Sheila looked frightened. She wasn't ready for decisions of that size as yet.

"You should," I said. "At least tell them that he is in the hospital, that the doctor suspects a heart attack, and that he's doing well—no complications or problems at present. They have the right to know."

"That's a good idea," she said, apparently relieved that the decision was made for her, then she took a deep breath. "When can I see Frank?"

"Right now," I smiled. "For five minutes."

"What about the rest of us?" Lisa asked.

"He should have no more than two visitors for ten minutes, every two hours. He's got to rest," I explained. "If you can wait another two hours, you can go in with Sheila the next time or perhaps your mother could go in with her. I think more than two visitors each time could be taxing."

"What about me?" asked Alex. He stood up very straight. "It's kind of tough, at the very beginning, for a cardiac patient to see his kids. Why don't we wait for a few days until your dad's out of CCU and in a regular hospital bed?"

"I'm not a kid," Alex said. "I'm going to be sixteen next month."

"I'm very grown up for my age," asserted Margot stoutly. "My teacher says so."

"I know you are, Margot," I said.

"So why can't we . . ."

"Listen, kids," Lisa interrupted. "You want your father to get well fast, don't you? So why don't you do what the doctor says?"

I didn't expect to have cause to be grateful to Lisa Mann but at that moment I was.

"Persons under sixteen aren't allowed in the Coronary Care Unit," I said, "but I'll arrange for you to see him as soon as he's moved to a regular hospital room in a couple of days." I turned to Sheila. "Let's go see the patient for a few minutes."

Actually, there was no need for me to escort her, but I

wanted to talk to her, privately. In her current state, the first sight of her spouse with all the tubes, wires, and devices hooked to him could easily crumple her barely held-together calm unless she was briefed beforehand.

"Sheila, when you see Frank lying there, you'll also see a bottle with clear liquid hung up and feeding into his arm by tube. That's just a glucose solution, which is running at a very slow rate. He'll be eating a diet low in fats, cholesterol, and salt, and he doesn't really need the nourishment from the glucose solution. But if we find we suddenly have to feed him some medicine intravenously, we don't have to waste time finding another vein and putting a new needle in him. Simple, huh?"

She nodded.

"Now about the other wires you'll see attached to him, there's the heart monitor—"

"It's all right, Doctor, *I* know what to expect. I watch all the hospital shows."

"That can help," I said, relieved.

"I just want to know how he is. Is he conscious?"

"Oh, yes. If he were asleep I'd tell you not to wake him but let him wake up by himself. But if he's awake, I should warn you, Sheila, that he might be angry."

"Angry? About what?"

"About having this happen to him. Some people take it that way—you know, sort of a 'Why does this happen to me?' attitude."

Sheila looked alarmed. "Isn't being angry bad for him?"

"It's a lot better than being scared. It might be his way of avoiding apprehension or fear. Anger can be very useful, you know. So if he lashes out at you, just take it, O.K.?"

It was the first time I'd seen her smile that day. "It'll be a pleasure, Doctor. Even if he beats me! He's alive!"

I escorted Sheila slowly past the other beds, with their array of paraphernalia, to let her get used to the otherworldly atmosphere. When we reached Frank's bed his head was back on his pillow, his eyes closed. The monitor showed a normal heart beat.

"He's asleep," I whispered to her. "Why don't you wait here until he . . ."

Frank's eyes suddenly opened. He looked at Sheila who looked back, pale and round-eyed, her lips trembling, a breath away from collapse.

"So," he said, trying to be stern, "who's minding the store?"

Sheila gave a trembling laugh. Wiping an eye, she stepped to the bed and gently took one hand in both hers. She kissed it and pressed it to her cheek. "I *told* you to take your rubbers this morning, didn't I?" Frank grinned weakly.

"Don't forget," I cautioned Sheila. "Five minutes." I headed back to the lounge.

"When I was a young girl," Sheila's mother sighed, "nobody had ever even heard of a coronary. Now everybody's dropping dead of it. You can't pick up a newspaper without reading about so and so dying of a coronary thrombosis. Why is that, Doctor?"

"It's very simple," Lisa answered for me. "Sixty or seventy years ago life was a lot simpler; it wasn't such a rat race. People weren't tense all the time, isn't that right, Doctor?"

I shrugged. "It's hard to say. Seems as though every generation thinks that the one before it had less to worry about. It may very well be. But, of course, sixty years ago there wasn't social security or unemployment benefits or hospitalization or welfare, and so they had a lot of things to worry about that we don't. On the other hand, doctors didn't know much about coronary ailments sixty years ago. It's possible, even probable, that when someone died of a coronary anywhere but in a hospital, the local physician ascribed it to acute indigestion or acute gall bladder trouble or an act of God. And you know the electrocardiograph machines weren't really in general use until the thirties. There may have been many more coronary deaths sixty years ago than were apparent in the vital statistics of that time."

"But people ate differently then, didn't they?" Lisa asked tenaciously. "I mean, nowadays we eat a lot more sweets and fatty things and that has a lot to do with the increasing heart trouble, doesn't it?"

"Yes," I agreed, "along with increased tension, heavier smoking, and so on, the change of diet to meats and sweets probably had a lot to do with it."

Lisa nodded smugly, glancing at her mother.

"But there's another major factor in the heart trouble epidemic that we can't do anything about," I added gravely.

"What's that?" Lisa asked, eager for some inside revelation.

"The medical profession itself." She looked at me uncomprehending. "We've found treatments for so many diseases that people are now living long enough to have heart trouble."

"Oh," she said grudgingly, "I never thought of that."

4. The Heart that Cured the Patient

"You're a dirty butcher!" Jane Bracken shrieked at Norman Sapphire, the cardiac surgeon I had brought into the case of her husband and my patient, Peter Bracken.

"You're going to kill my father!" shrilled her normally sweet-tempered daughter Rose.

As Norman Sapphire later related to me, he didn't lose his aplomb even though this unusually loud presurgical conference was going on in the waiting room of Cedars Hospital's Cardiac Intensive Care section, where everything could be heard by patient visitors. He had had enough family conferences to appreciate the intense feelings involved.

Peter Bracken, a man of fifty-nine, had checked into the hospital that morning. He was suffering from near blockage of both coronary arteries and was an imminent candidate for a massive coronary, which could be fatal. His only hope, Norman had just explained to the family—Mrs. Bracken, her daughter Rose, and son Martin, a pediatrician—lay in immediate coronary artery bypass operation. He carefully pointed out the mortality rate in this open-heart surgery procedure and the odds for Peter's recovery, given his current state of health.

"All right," an agonized Mrs. Bracken exclaimed, "but whatever you do, Dr. Sapphire, please don't tell him he's going to be operated on."

"He's got to be told," Norm replied. "He's sound of mind. It's *his* heart. He's got to know all the odds, to make the final decision. After all, *he* has to sign a release."

"I'll sign for him. Please, let me," pleaded his daughter. "If my father found out what's going to be done to him he'd die before the operation."

"You don't know what a nervous type he is, Dr. Sapphire," her mother added. "If he gets the slightest idea, he'll go to pieces."

"I'm sorry," Norm said gently, "but he'll have to be told. Don't worry. We won't frighten him."

As a children's doctor, his father's problems were well out of Martin Bracken's province, but he was caught up in the fever of father-protecting. "Doctor Sapphire, I don't think he should be told. I mean, my father is hypersensitive. He's always suffered from a nervous stomach . . ."

"You don't mean to say you're going to tell him about this dreadful operation," Jane Bracken gasped.

"You're not actually going to tell my father his chances of survival are . . ."

"I'm not going to be the one doing that," Norm said, with, I suspect, some sense of relief. "Dr. Karpman will. But I'm afraid your father's going to have to be told everything.

A patient who has to make the decision about his operation . . ."

"We'll make the decision," Rose said tearfully. "Let me sign for my father."

". . . is entitled to know everything about the operation he's to undergo," Norm continued. "After all, he's in full possession of his faculties, he's a grown man—"

It was at this point that the Bracken woman started hurling their invective.

The seeds of this drama had been planted nine years before when Peter Bracken, a small pleasant-mannered man, first came to see me on the recommendation of a friend who was one of my patients. His wife, a handsome woman, slightly taller than he, accompanied him. She followed him into my office as though it were the most ordinary thing in the world for a wife to be present throughout her husband's medical consultation with his doctor.

"My heart stops," he told me. "Every now and then it just stops."

His wife nodded vigorously.

Anxiety was written all over his face. His fingers, with well-bitten nails, plucked nervously at his trouser leg.

"For how long a period does your heart stop?"

"At least a minute," his wife said.

"An *entire* minute, Mr. Bracken?"

"Maybe half a minute," he said grudgingly. "I'll have twelve, fifteen regular beats then the heart stops, then another twelve, fifteen regular beats, then it stops again."

"Instead of saying your heart stops, could you describe it as your heart skips beats?"

Bracken's eyes sought his wife's. She nodded.

"Yes," he said thoughtfully. "I guess you could say my heart is skipping beats, although when I'm waiting for that one after the skipped one, it seems to take forever."

"He gets so upset, Doctor," his wife interjected.

"It's a psychological reaction," I said. "Waiting for your heartbeat to return after a delayed beat can make a few seconds seem like a half minute or even a minute. Most people, you know, have occasional missed beats."

"But he's so nervous to begin with, Doctor."

"Tell me about that delayed beat, Mr. Bracken. When it finally comes, is it a strong beat, a weak one, or the same as the ones before it?"

"Oh, it's very strong. You know, *thump*—like it's slapping the inside of my chest."

"What does it feel like?"

"Well, it sounds awfully ridiculous . . ."

"He says that late beat feels like his heart is turning over in his chest," Mrs. Bracken interrupted.

"That's not ridiculous," I said. "It's a very common sensation with missed heartbeats."

"You see, dear?" said Mrs. Bracken. Bracken continued to look at me with frightened eyes. Then, unexpectedly, he yawned.

"How long do these heart-skip spells go on, Mr. Bracken?"

"Half hour. Sometimes an hour."

"What do you mean, Peter?" Mrs. Bracken said. "Sometimes they go on for hours. Remember last week?"

"Sometimes they go on for hours," her husband repeated to me.

"Do these spells happen every day?"

"Almost. Sometimes they'll stop for a day or two, then start again."

"Does it happen on work days?"

"Both. Work days and weekends," Mrs. Bracken said.

"What sort of work do you do, Mr. Bracken?"

"We're in the selling business," his wife said. "We sell notions and novelties in supermarkets. We replenish every week."

Bracken yawned again.

"You must be tired, Mr. Bracken."

"Of course he's tired, ever since this thing started with his heart."

"Are these heart spells interfering with your sleep, Mr. Bracken?"

He hesitated. "Yes."

"Tell him the truth, Peter."

He sighed. "To tell you the truth, Doctor, I'm afraid to go to sleep. I'm always afraid I'm not going to wake up."

"Now that's ridiculous," I said.

"He's morbid," his wife said. "Always afraid something terrible is going to happen to him. I've always been the strong one. I had a kidney removed six years ago, and I wasn't afraid for one minute that I was going to die. But Peter won't even go up in an airplane. He's always afraid of disaster."

Bracken looked at me solemnly. " 'A throe upon the features. A hurry in the breath. An Ecstacy of parting. Denominated Death.' "

"What?"

"Emily Dickinson," he said.

"He's always quoting poetry," his wife said, adoringly. "He reads poetry every chance he gets. Poe, Shakespeare . . ."

"William Cullen Bryant, Robert Browning, John Keats," Peter added, "but Emily Dickinson is my favorite. I love her poems."

"Good," I said. "You take a book of her poetry to bed tonight and read yourself to sleep and stop worrying about not waking up. I'm going to put you through a thorough physical examination and get some tests after we're done here. My feeling is that these sensations you're having are due to extra beats of the heart which come a little earlier than the normal beat. They're called extrasystoles or extra beats. Systole is Greek for 'pulling together' or 'contracting.' When your heart pumps, it contracts, forcing the blood forward, and you can sometimes feel it as a heartbeat. No one has ever been known to die of infrequent extrasystoles, awake or asleep. They're probably harmless."

"My heart stops and you say it's harmless?"

"Your heart doesn't stop. It's only having a premature beat. The heart is a series of four chambers. Each chamber is supposed to fill up with blood before it contracts and squirts it all into the next chamber or into the major artery. Sometimes, however, a chamber does a premature beat while it's still filling up, and the next chamber gets only a fraction of its full capacity for blood. It's frequently the fourth chamber, the left ventricle. So it holds off on its contraction until it gets the next load. That is, it simply waits. That's why you think your heart has stopped. Then when it again starts pumping into the main artery leading from the heart, the aorta, it regains its regular beats right in rhythm again."

Bracken nodded.

"Your heart is like the engine in a car. What keeps the chambers in the heart pumping in proper sequence are like spark plugs buried in the muscle walls which trigger each chamber in turn by electric sparks. Sometimes a spark plug misfires. These spark plugs, which are called the pacemakers . . ."

"I thought pacemakers were batteries that are put into people with bad hearts," Mrs. Bracken said.

"I'm talking about natural pacemakers. The other kind are electronic pacemakers, which are implanted under the skin and hooked to the heart by an electric wire wormed through a vein. They're used to help keep the heart chambers pumping if the natural pacemakers fall down on the job."

Bracken turned pale. "Will I need one?"

"Absolutely not. There's nothing wrong with your natural pacemakers."

"But you said one of them is misfiring."

"No, I said it was *like* a spark plug in a car engine misfiring. You see, there are hundreds of nerve tissue bits in the chamber walls that are reserve pacemakers. They are supposed to go into action only if the major pacemakers should fail to spark a contraction of a chamber in time. Occasionally, one of these reserve pacemakers may go out of sync and start firing on its own. It's a normal occurrence for almost everybody now and then. That's that little premature contraction every fifteenth beat, that little heart skip. Unless it's frequent or repetitious, then it's not a serious form of arrhythmia to have."

"What's arrhythmia?"

"Lovely, musical word, isn't it?" I thought that might touch the poet in Bracken. "Arrhythmia means out of rhythm. Any variation from the normal beat of the heart."

"And I've got arrhythmia?" Bracken didn't look happy.

"A very mild form. If arrhythmia was a respiratory ailment, for instance, you would have the sniffles."

"How long will it go on?" Mrs. Bracken asked.

"Hard to say. Might go away in a manner of minutes, might hang on for years. Might come back. A lot of people are discovered to have it at some time in their lives. A few are born with it. Some develop it late in life."

"What causes it?" asked Mrs. Bracken.

"Could come from too much coffee, tiredness or worry, cigarette smoking. Do you smoke?"

"Not anymore," said Mrs. Bracken with finality. "Starting right now."

Bracken nodded meekly.

"I should have given it up a long time ago."

"Does this heart skipping run in families?" his wife asked. "Peter's mother had the same thing, didn't she, dear?"

"Oh, hers was much worse," said Peter. "Her heart used to get going like a machine gun. She was positive each time she was going to die. She'd cry and go to bed and always say she was surprised to find herself alive in the morning."

I wondered how much Peter's childhood had to do with his present anxieties.

"Your mother probably had another form of arrhythmia," I said. "For example, in one arrhythmia called paroxysmal atrial tachycardia, suddenly the heart starts beating at a tremendous pace, often accompanied by breathlessness. It can be caused by one of the reserve pacemakers I described. Only instead of firing every fifteenth or sixteenth beat, it starts firing nonstop at a rapid rate and the chambers that pump the blood into the system start pumping at two or even three times the normal rate. It's usually not dangerous if it goes on for just a few hours, or even for a day or two. But in some people the heart can start to fatigue or get tired after awhile. Nowadays it's pretty easy to control with drugs and sedatives."

"My mother never used anything," Peter said mournfully. "In those days nobody did. She would just lie down till it stopped."

"I'm sure that helped, too. Paroxysmal tachycardia often results from fatigue or tension, or irritation or worry."

"Are you sure that what I've got is harmless?" Bracken asked.

"We'll start finding out right now." I reached for a yellow pad and pencil. "We'll start with your history."

The most significant item in Bracken's medical history was that he had suffered a nervous stomach as a youth, and had received an army medical discharge during World War II as a result. The symptoms diminished when he learned that they stemmed from anxiety.

When Bracken answered questions about his medical history, he repeatedly looked at Mrs. Bracken for corroboration.

"All right now," I said cheerfully, standing up, "shall we start on your tests?"

To my surprise Mrs. Bracken followed us into the examination room and stayed through all the tests: blood pressure reading, resting EKG, stress cardiogram on the treadmill, x-rays, blood tests, the general physical checkup. When I asked Bracken to remove his pants for a hernia and prostate check, however, I asked her to look away. Somehow, it seemed the right thing to do.

A few days later I reviewed the test results with the Brackens. His heart, I said, was in excellent running order.

"Oh, Doctor, you've made me the happiest woman in the world," Mrs. Bracken said.

" 'Faith is a fine invention, when gentlemen can see! But microscopes are prudent, in an emergency,' " Peter said, beaming. "Emily Dickinson."

"He loves poetry," said Mrs. Bracken proudly.

A few weeks later, she phoned me to say that Peter's heart condition had subsided. She thanked me extravagantly. From her reaction, one would think that I had saved Bracken's life simply by telling them his heart skips were relatively harmless. She said also that he had given up cigarettes. That could do nothing but help.

Two years after that, Mrs. Bracken phoned me to tell me her husband had heart pains that very morning. They had been of very short duration, and in fact he was well enough to come on the extension phone in their apartment as we talked.

"We got into the car to drive to a new supermarket. Peter was just going to put his foot on the starter. All of a sudden he felt so weak he told me he thought he would faint."

"I had these chest pains," Bracken said. "I couldn't catch my breath."

"Tell him about your heartbeat, Peter. It was racing, Doctor."

"It was beating very fast and hard, Doctor."

I asked him if he had ever had this combination of symptoms before. He hadn't. I asked them to come in to my office but Bracken was not to drive himself. They came in a cab. I whisked him into an examination room, his wife right behind me.

I took his pulse, blood pressure, examined the interior of his eyes with an ophthalmoscope to inspect the small blood vessels. I looked at his fingers and toes to see if his circulation was normal. I examined his chest and listened to his heart with a stethoscope.

As I checked him over, I encouraged them to talk about their occupation. Their business, it seems, had taken a drop. Two of the supermarkets they sold to had closed. That morning when the symptoms had occurred the Brackens had been heading for a new supermarket to see if they could establish a notions and novelty stand there. Interestingly, when we talked about their business Mrs. Bracken let her husband do all the talking. I inquired idly about the supermarket manager they were going to meet for the first time that day. He had a reputation for being tough, Bracken told me.

I finally put away my stethoscope. "You can put your pants and shirt back on, Mr. Bracken, and I'll see both of you in my office."

I told them there was no indication of a heart attack. They both looked more surprised than relieved.

"But the chest pains . . ." said Bracken.

"The way Peter was breathing in the car this morning and his heart was racing, Doctor, it must have been a heart attack."

"There are a number of illnesses that imitate all the symptoms of heart disease," I told them. "A gall bladder attack, for instance, has a great resemblance to a coronary . . ."

"You mean it's his gall bladder?" She put a hand on Bracken's arm. His eyes were round.

"No, that was just an example of the kind of disorder that fools people into thinking they have heart trouble. A lot of things can cause chest pains. For instance, a pain can come from within the chest wall itself, entirely divorced from the heart. That's called neurocirculatory asthenia. Some people with nervous dispositions or under tension have headaches, others have chest pains. So chest pains themselves do not mean a heart attack. Neither does shortness of breath or palpitations. Even indigestion can resemble cardiac pain.

"He had a very light breakfast," she protested. "I mean, with his stomach, I'm so careful."

"It wasn't indigestion, Mrs. Bracken. I'm just going through all of these for your benefit so in the future you don't get frightened needlessly. It's estimated there are up to twenty million people in this country who think they have heart trouble, act accordingly and yet don't have it. Bursitis in the shoulder is mistaken for it. An inflammation of your esophagus or your intestines can give you the symptoms of a coronary. Even a hernia can fool a patient or doctors . . ."

"Peter has a double hernia, Doctor . . ."

"No, I don't mean the ones down there. That's called an inguinal hernia. I mean one that can pop up through a small hole in the diaphragm muscle between the stomach and the lungs, a hiatus hernia."

"What do you think it was with me, Doctor?"

"Nervous tension. You were going to a new market this morning. You were going to try and sell to a manager you had never met before who had a reputation for being tough."

"Of course, that's what it was, Peter. You remember last night you couldn't sleep from worrying about today's meeting."

Bracken stared at me. "You mean to tell me just from nerves I can have all these chest pains and my heart can beat a mile a minute and I can have trouble catching my breath?"

"During World War I," I told him, "many soldiers in England were discharged as heart cases. They showed the same symptoms you did. It was called soldier's heart. They went home and lived like invalids. Years later when we knew more about the heart, it was realized that all they suffered from was the same thing you had today—chest pains due to nervous tension."

Bracken smiled unexpectedly. "We've come a long way, Doctor, haven't we?"

"In cardiology, yes."

Despite all reassurances, the Brackens kept returning over the years for what he was sure, at each time, was a sudden heart attack. Bracken never drove in for these examinations. Either he and his wife arrived by taxicab or his son, then a fledgling pediatrician, and later his daughter, drove them in. Both children showed their father the same compassionate devotion their mother did. It reminded me of a sophomore intellectual during bull sessions in my undergraduate days who maintained that the reason God had been invented was not so much out of our need to feel protected as our need to find someone to protect. That thesis was certainly substantiated by watching the Brackens in action.

Most of the symptoms could be traced to anxieties which flourished easily in his piano-wire personality. He had become a cardiac neurotic, aware of every heartbeat, every twinge in the chest. One time he had a rib inflammation that mimicked the shooting pains of a coronary thrombosis. On another occasion, he was rushed to my office when he complained of dizziness and pounding heart, and it developed he had been in a depressed mood and had simply hyperventilated from all the deep sighs and rapid breathing. Treatment was simple. I told him next time to breathe into a paper bag or even simply hold his breath; that would build up enough carbon dioxide into his blood system to restore a balance with oxygen.

Once, Mrs. Bracken privately apologized to me for the many times her husband had come in with false alarms.

"I suppose Peter is really a hypochondriac."

"The greater difference between a hypochondriac and the rest of us," I told her, "is that the hypochondriac is scared and admits it." I said I would rather have patients who ran to me with every suspicion of heart ailment than those who suppressed their fears and went on with business as usual.

The visits began to drop off, but the phone calls came regularly, and they followed the same general pattern. "Hello, Doctor, this is Peter Bracken. I hate to bother you, Doctor, but this morning when I got up . . ." and then would come the detailed description of a tingling of the fingers of his left hand followed by shooting pains through his shoulder (he had been sleeping on his left side with his arm cramped under him) or the report that his face was flushed and his heart pounding (he had had too much coffee). It was always some variation on one theme—his heart was sending out a final distress signal before its imminent collapse. His shaky voice always seemed to indicate he was trying to steel himself for the inevitable without too much success. I would suggest the innocuous causes for his symptoms, tell him to wait a few hours and phone me if the symptoms didn't clear up, he would thank me with a dubious note in his voice, and that would be the end of it for the time being.

Then came one morning the familiar "I'm sorry to bother you . . ." but the tone of his voice wasn't familiar. It was the voice of a man trying to keep genuine fears in check. He told me his symptoms in a voice that trembled only once or twice.

"I started feeling pains down the sides of my chest in the middle of the night . . . from my shoulders right down to my lower ribs . . . No, they're not getting worse . . . No, they don't hurt terribly, but they just won't go away."

"Are there any other symptoms?"

There was a pause. "I just have this feeling that I'm going to die."

Despite all his deeply rooted hypochondria, Bracken had never quite said anything like that. It's not uncommon for people to feel a pervasive sense of imminent disaster at the beginning of a heart attack.

My intuitive feeling was that this time Peter Bracken was not crying wolf. He actually might be having a coronary.

"Mr. Bracken," I said as casually as I could, "it's hard to tell over the telephone, but this could be a minor heart spasm. I'll tell you what. I'm on my way over to the West Hospital to see a patient. Why don't you have someone run you over to the emergency room there and we'll get a cardiogram and I'll check you over."

Actually, I was not on my way to see a patient anywhere. It was my so-called day off, and I was catching up on paperwork in my office. But if Bracken had thought I was making a special trip to the hospital to see him, he would have been beside himself with anxiety.

When I arrived in the emergency room of the hospital, I saw a small, flurried clump of people near the nurse's station. In the center were Peter Bracken, still dressed, and his wife. The nurse had asked Bracken to go into the examination room, and Mrs. Bracken had felt it was her inalienable right to accompany him. The rules of the hospital, however, were quite rigid. Family members were not allowed to be present during a patient's examination, but Bracken had refused to go into the examination room without his wife. I got the head nurse to bend the hospital's rule sufficiently to let her in. The son and daughter remained in the waiting room.

A preliminary examination indicated that Bracken was suffering a coronary occlusion. His systolic blood pressure had dropped slightly, his EKG demonstrated a definite myocardial infarction. I had him transferred to the hospital's Coronary Care Unit.

In the case of a minor heart attack, a firm scar will usually form with little outside help, and once formed, it will be stronger than the heart tissue around it. In a short time, if there were no complications, Bracken would be out of the hospital.

Considering his long-standing history of profound anxiety, Bracken took everything fairly well. He had been rigid with fear when I met him in the hospital prior to the examination, but he perked up a bit when I got there. Most people find the arrival of their doctor itself a kind of balm. Once he was transferred to the Cardiac Care Unit, he was sedated long enough to allow him to adjust to his new environment, and the sense of being cared for with unflagging concern had a pacifying, relaxing effect.

Bracken had an extraordinarily smooth convalescence. He was pain-free after twenty-four hours and, after four days he was transferred from Coronary Care to a coronary observation ward. By the end of the second week he was sitting up in a chair and being readied to return home.

But an hour after lunch on the fifteenth day, he suddenly developed a pallor, a faint chest depression, and a feeling of lightheadedness. I was called to the hospital and found him perspiring profusely. An EKG demonstrated increasing heart strain. It was obvious that his coronary insufficiency had become worse. It appeared that the relatively minor infarction that he had just passed through was now threatening to become a massive heart attack. It began to appear that

Bracken might be a candidate for coronary artery bypass surgery.

To find the exact location of the coronary artery narrowing was going to require angiocardiography, a procedure by which the heart chambers and the blood vessels can be studied by introducing a catheter, a long thin, flexible tube through an artery in the arm or the groin and threaded back to the chambers of the heart. Once the end of the catheter has been maneuvered to the desired location in the heart or to the base of each coronary artery, a harmless contrasting dye is injected via the tube. Motion picture x-rays and videotapes are then recorded to study the function of the heart chambers and, more importantly, to define the degree and location of any narrowing or obstruction in the coronary arteries.

Use of this ingenious diagnostic procedure has multiplied in the comparatively few years since its introduction in 1967 and techniques are constantly being improved. But, as with any surgical procedure, no matter how minor, small risks exist, and therefore before patients can be put through this procedure their written consent must be obtained.

Normally in angiocardiography the patient has plenty of time to discuss it with the doctor and surgeon, to get adjusted to the idea of having an incision made in an arm or a groin and a catheter threaded back into the heart. Any initial resistence to the idea is also generally overcome if the patient's feeling of well-being has been eroded to the point where he or she is likely to agree to something that has a risk, even if only minimal, if it will eventually help him.

In the case of Peter Bracken we didn't have the time to coax him into a suitable frame of mind. It was too sudden an emergency.

First I advised the patient be moved from the small hospital to a major hospital equipped with the most sophisticated surgery facilities. Needless to say, Mrs. Bracken sat in the van next to his stretcher the entire trip.

I called in a cardiologist, Dr. Mel Wilder, to perform the coronary arteriogram, not only because of his excellent reputation but because he had had intensive training in the manipulation of the kind of catheter that would be needed in this particular case. I saw to it that he had the opportunity to explain the angiographic procedure to Bracken alone in his new hospital room. I explained the same facts to the rest of the Bracken family in the waiting room.

"How risky is it, Doctor?" Mrs. Bracken asked anxiously.

"About as much, say, as in a blood transfusion."

No one appeared relieved. I recalled that among other prejudices, Peter was allergic to the sight of blood.

"Or having an appendix or tonsils removed," I amended, hurriedly.

"Will you do the angiogram?" his daughter asked me.

I shook my head. "No, you've got to have a cardiologist with special training in cardiac catherization," I explained. "That's why I've called in Dr. Wilder to handle it. Remember, there is no pain with it except for the initial needle stick when the local anesthetic is put in the arm or in the groin, just like when the gums are numbed by the dentist before he starts to work on your teeth."

"You'll be there during the operation, Doctor, won't you?" Mrs. Bracken looked at me imploringly.

"It's not an operation, just a procedure. Of course I'll be there, unless I'm called away in an emergency. But Dr. Wilder will actually do the catheterization and is extraordinarily competent to handle any complications."

"How can you expect Peter to go through that thing

without you being there?" she asked, "I don't even think you can get him to do it *with* you but without you!" There was almost horror in her eyes.

"But I just told you," I said wearily, "that I *will* be there unless an emergency comes up."

As it happened an emergency *did* come up, and I had to be elsewhere during the angiogram procedure.

Fortunately, Peter Bracken showed enough confidence in Mel Wilder to go through with it. It may have been the doctor's persuasive manner or the after-effects of Peter's last sedation or his general sense of demoralization, but there was less resistance than anticipated.

Mel's phone call to me after he had performed the angiogram was not encouraging.

"Both coronary arteries are almost totally blocked, Harold." he said. "Left ninety-eight percent. Right, ninety-five percent. It's up there on the TV monitor."

"What about the x-ray film for confirmation?"

"They'll be developed in twenty minutes. But there's no question. Ninety-eight percent and ninety-five percent."

The wonder of human design! With one segment of a vital pipeline narrowed to only two percent of capacity, the other five percent, Peter Bracken's circulatory system was still functioning and Bracken was living, breathing, speaking, thinking. The urgent question was how long the miracle would sustain before a massive coronary or a ventricular fibrillation or heart failure brought everything to a halt.

Time was of the essence. We agreed on the phone that Bracken's only chance lay in an immediate bypass operation of both coronary arteries. I would return to the hospital as soon as possible and try to get Bracken's immediate consent to the double bypass. In the meantime I directed that Doctor Sapphire, a noted cardiac surgeon, be alerted. He would check the motion picture x-rays and reserve an operation room. He would also brief the Bracken family, still in the waiting room, on everything that had been happening.

It was during that briefing that Mrs. Bracken and her daughter became so emotionally carried away that they began shouting names.

I came back just about this time and the Brackens turned to me with the relief of victims beleagured by a dragon welcoming a knight on horseback—only to discover that the knight was in league with the dragon.

"You can't tell him, Dr. Karpman!" pleaded Mrs. Bracken, dissolving in tears. "You know he won't be able to take it!"

The only reassurance I could give her was to let her accompany Norm and me to her husband's bedside, on condition that she keep a cheerful countenance and say nothing.

"Peter," I said to the wan, apathetic figure in the hospital bed—it was the first time I'd called him by his first name in all those years—"I want to congratulate you. The way you agreed to that angiogram without a single objection. Dr. Sapphire here can tell you how many hours it sometimes takes to persuade people to permit the coronary angiogram to be performed. With you it took—how many minutes? Maybe two?"

"People are afraid of it?" Bracken had lost some of his apathy.

"Peter," I said, "I had a male patient half your age—big, strapping fellow, too. I had to encourage him for two days to have an angiogram. He was plain scared. I was really impressed with you."

"Well, it wasn't much." He beamed.

"The way it stands now, Peter, your angiogram shows a great deal of blockage in both your main right coronary artery and your left one. Dr. Sapphire and I are agreed that he should proceed immediately with what's called a saphenous vein bypass. In this case, it would take at least two grafts, maybe three."

"Peter," Norm added, "we've reviewed the angiograms and they show that you are one of the fortunate ones who can have a heart operation that will most likely prevent a major heart attack, which now seems to be developing. You are a lucky man. If those arteries had been too badly diseased, we wouldn't have been able to offer you an operation, and we would have had to sit tight hoping it didn't get any worse. The chances of your getting worse without an operation are quite enormous, but the chances of you being improved with an operation are over ninety percent. So you've got the odds all on your side."

I described the operation briefly. Removal of segments of the saphenous vein from his leg. Opening the chest and grafting on the needed vein sections from the aorta, where blood, freshly oxygenated from the lungs, is then piped via the vein to just beyond the atherosclerosis-blocked sections of the coronary arteries. As I touched on the salient points I could see Norm, out of the corner of my eye, half-supporting Mrs. Bracken, who looked ill.

"What do you think my chances are, Doctor?" Bracken asked in a surprisingly strong, steady voice.

"I think they're excellent," I answered. "Coronary conditions aside, you're in excellent shape for your age. Your weight's good, the rest of your heart is healthy. A major myocardial infarction has not occurred. I think your chances are better than good."

"And you think I should have the operation?"

"We both think so, the doctor and I, and as soon as possible."

"Well, that's good enough for me. The sooner the better."

As I recall it, Mrs. Bracken burst out with something to the effect that perhaps Peter should think it over first.

He looked at her. "What is there to think about?" he said irritably. "Every time you go to a doctor you put your life in his hands. After nine years with the same one, why should I hold back now?"

As he was being prepared for the operation, Bracken looked up at me. " 'Surgeons must be very careful, when they take the knife, Underneath their fine incisions, Stirs the culprit—Life!' Emily Dickinson."

The operation was a greater success than anybody had anticipated. The major myocardial infarction was avoided, his heart functioned better and so did Peter Bracken. It may have been the knowledge that in the face of his crisis, he was the one the family who had unexpectedly shown the most calm, the least trepidation, that gave him his new found sense of security.

A lot of his hypochondria has vanished, he no longer frets endlessly over small annoyances and worries, he takes brisk, hour-long walks twice a day, he thinks nothing now of taking trips by air. When he runs into other post-operative caridacs and exchanges stories of hospital experiences with them, they often say admiringly, "My, I wish I had your courage." His answer is often couched in the brief words of a poet other than Emily Dickinson. He quotes William Shakespeare from *King John:* "Courage mounteth with occasion."

5. How to Match a Miracle

Ten days after he had been admitted to the hospital, Frank Justin was already sitting up in an upholstered armchair, in pajamas and bathrobe, reading a book when I walked into the room.

"Good morning, Frank."

"Morning, Doc." He dog-eared the page, put the book on top of a stack on his night table, and gave me his usual opening self-diagnosis: "I'm doing fine, huh?"

"Ten days after a coronary and you're out of bed and sitting in a chair? One of us must be doing something right. How do you feel?"

"Fantastic."

"That's understandable. Your temperature's back to normal. Your cardiogram gives no indication of any complications in your heart beat. Your cardiac rhythm is steady as a rock. Remember what I told you that first day in the Coronary Care Unit?"

"What?"

"I said if your recovery was really good—"

"... I'd be out in three weeks. Sure, I remember."

"Well, you've run ahead of my estimate. You're in great shape. So good that instead of staying here eleven more days, you'll be going home within the week."

"Why can't I go home today?"

Before I'd walked into the room, I'd known Frank was going to give me a hard time. The feeling didn't come from any medical sixth sense. It came from the fact that Frank had given me a hard time from the day of his first phone call.

"You can't go home yet. You're not well enough."

He looked at me almost with indignation. "You just told me I'm in great shape."

"In great shape for the end of your tenth day of recovery."

"And I *feel* in great shape, so I must be well enough!"

Years ago, Frank had quit school, had borrowed six hundred dollars, and plunged into the garment business, investing in a line of playsuits that seasoned manufacturers told him was a dog. He came out with a profit and great confidence in his own unorthodox judgment, which continued to be vindicated in his business career. People who have worked their way up by pitting themselves against established authority in their field tend to distrust established authority in other fields. For physicians this isn't necessarily bad; they often find their skill in communication getting a good workout when they're dealing with feisty patients.

"*Feeling* well enough and *being* well enough aren't necessarily the same thing," I told Frank. "Right now, it's like the good feeling you have when you *stop* hitting yourself on the head with a hammer. After the pain and the shock, your convalescence is like putting down the hammer. You feel fantastic, but it's not a good measure of—"

". . . how well I am," he finished. "Look, I know myself, and the way I feel right now, lying in a hospital is a complete waste of time."

"So you've been telling me every day."

"If I'm being a nuisance, that seems to be the only way I can get my point across."

"Actually, I don't mind your being a nuisance."

He blinked. "You're kidding."

"No, I'm serious. I've seen patients physically recover from a coronary as fast as you, but their psychological recuperation wasn't always as quick. A lot of people treat themselves like invalids long after their hearts have healed. But I don't think that's going to be your problem."

"The only problem I got is that I'm wasting my time here," Frank retorted.

"You're thinking of your business, aren't you?"

"*One* of the things I'm thinking about!"

My voice throbbed with synthetic compassion. "Here you are in the hospital and none of your competitors are."

That reached him. He gave me a sheepish grin. "Yeah. How about that?"

"And then there's all that tennis you're missing."

"And that's another thing. I had to drop out of a tournament on account of you rushing me in here."

"Can you find it in your healing heart to forgive me?"

"If you don't let it happen again."

I dropped the bantering tone. "That's why I'm keeping you in the hospital. So it won't happen again."

"I could be convalescing at home," Frank persisted.

"You will be, in good time."

"You call this good time? I call it wasted time."

"Do you really miss your office that much?"

"I miss it and I miss tennis. I miss everything!"

"What about your wife and family?"

"Why should I miss them? Sheila's here every day, and the kids are here every other day."

"You probably see more of them here in the hospital than you did at home."

He looked like I'd kicked him. "Now, come on, Harold, that's a low blow and no way to talk to a sick man."

"At least it proves that being in the hospital isn't a complete waste of time, doesn't it?"

Frank looked out of the window. "It doesn't prove a thing."

I wondered if any of the buyers Frank sold to were as tough as he was being right then. I sat down in the visitor's chair. "Frank, I told you your bounce back has been tremendous and your psychological recovery's even ahead of your physical recovery. But there can be too much of a good thing. Sometimes that self-confidence is caused by the wish to just forget about the coronary altogether. I've had patients who've gone through pretty much what you have who've absolutely denied they had had a heart attack at all."

"Oh, I don't deny it. I know I had those chest pains and tired feelings and all that. If you and the hospital say it was a heart attack, I take your word for it."

"Thanks, we appreciate that," I said straight-faced. "You know, in the ten days you've been here, you haven't once asked what brought the attack on."

He shrugged. "Hell, I was pushing too hard. Working too much, spreading myself too thin."

"Maybe it wasn't the amount of work but the *way* you've been working."

"Oh?" He thought a moment and shrugged. "I don't know. I work about the way everybody else in the business works. Some of them work a lot harder than me. Some get coronaries but a lot of them don't."

"Did you ever think that some people are coronary prone?"

"Really? You mean there's a type that has heart attacks and a type that doesn't?"

"A lot of doctors are beginning to think so."

"No kidding? Someone ought to write a book about it." His tone was a shade too guileless, but I bit.

"Two well-known cardiologists have. A book called—"

". . . *Type A Behavior and Your Heart,*" Frank rattled off, snatching a book off the nightstand and holding it up. He loved this kind of coup. "By Meyer Friedman, M.D. and Ray H. Rosenman, M.D. I've set myself to read a heart book a day. I've only got thirty pages to go."

"Well! You really *haven't* been wasting your time, have you? What do you think of it?"

"I'm inclined to think they're right. I mean, people running around with a lot of stresses and anxieties . . . sure, they're more likely to have heart attacks. You know, when I think of it, my business is full of Type A people."

"Would you say I'm looking at one right now?"

Frank blinked. "Me? Hell, no. I mean, I don't deny I've got stress and tension in my life, but I know people who have a hell of a lot more who don't drop in their tracks."

"It's not the amount of stress one is subject to, it's—"

". . . how you handle the stress. Yeah, I read that. Well, I think I happen to handle it pretty damn well."

"So do a lot of Type A's."

"And so do a lot of Type B's," Frank said, "so what makes you think I'm not a Type B?"

"Well, let's look at Type A types. First of all, they live by the clock. Never enough hours in the day for all the things they want to get done."

"Well, I'm not that way. I just happen to hate the idea of wasting time."

"Like when you're behind a slow driver?"

"Everybody hates a slow driver. I give them the horn."

"What about waiting for a table in a restaurant? You can't honk a horn there."

"I can walk out. Even with a reservation, if the head-waiter says there's going to be a wait, I walk."

"Even if the food is great?"

"Oh, food doesn't mean that much to me. I think all that gourmet stuff is overrated . . ."

"You mean it's a waste of time."

"We-ell . . ."

"Tell me, if your wife cooks at home and the house-keeper is off, have you ever done the dishes?"

"Say, what's with all these questions?"

"To show you what type you are. Type A's live by the clock. They can't stand driving behind a slow car or having to wait in line for anything. They hate doing trivial things like adding up check stubs or doing the dishes. It's all in the book you've been reading today, the part you've already been through. Didn't you read it?"

"Well, actually I sort of skimmed it."

"Typical Type A behavior. Those people skim through books. They even skim through *condensations* of books, because the most important thing to them—"

". . . is saving time, I know."

"That's another characteristic of Type A."

"What?"

"They finish sentences for you."

Frank looked mortified.

"And they drive hard at everything. Like quote, 'I've set myself to reading one heart book a day.' "

He grinned. "Guess I should of said 'skimming,' not 'reading.' O.K., maybe I do live by the clock and maybe I do push kind of hard. But, hell, I'm in a highly competitive business. Dog eat dog. I've got a million problems on my head and every minute I'm thinking of them. When I'm reading, when I'm eating, when I'm on the john . . ."

"And you don't think you're a Type A? Know what 'polyphasic thinking' is?"

He nodded. "Yeah, that I remember from the book. Polyphasic thinking is when you think of two or three different things even when you're doing something else entirely different. But like I said, I'm in a dog-eat-dog business. Got to be on your toes every minute. I stop competing I might as well give up soft goods and take up . . . well, how about cardiology?"

I nodded. "Yes, there are plenty of Type A doctors. Maybe that's why I know what I'm talking about. Look, I'm not asking you to stop competing. After all, Type A people aren't the only ones who have to compete for a living. What did you read about Type B's?"

"Type B's?" His brows knit. "Oh, yeah. They're the ones who know how to relax, how to enjoy, and all that crap."

" 'All that crap' is what keeps them from having coronaries. A lot of research," I pointed at the book in his hands, "seems to confirm the fact that people with an anxiety abou time, who find their principal joy in competing at everything, who can't relax or enjoy leisure, are two and a half times more prone to heart attacks than—"

". . . people who can relax and enjoy leisure—oops, I finished your sentence."

I couldn't help smiling.

"Frank, Type B people obviously have to compete at work, too. They can have a million problems, but they try to solve them one at a time. They concentrate on what they're doing wholeheartedly. When they leave work, they leave the problems and competing at work. When they sit down to dinner, they enjoy the dinner wholeheartedly. They enjoy their family wholeheartedly. When they play games, they enjoy them wholeheartedly. Maybe that's why their hearts stay whole so much longer than Type A's."

"Listen, Doc, I don't need this lecture. Hell, I know how to enjoy wholeheartedly. Why do you think I like tennis so much?"

"Why?"

"Because I enjoy playing it wholeheartedly."

"I would say you enjoy *winning* wholeheartedly. That's why you're always in tournaments, right?"

"Is that a sin?"

"If winning is the most important thing about your playing, yes."

"Are you trying to tell me Type B people don't enjoy winning?"

"Everybody enjoys winning, but when Type B people play, they realize their school days are over, they're not on the college team; and when they lose, they can still enjoy having played. Playing to win, playing to beat someone else, is just incidental. Playing for enjoyment of the sport and for sharing that enjoyment with other people is what you're going to have to learn, Frank. End of lecture."

He settled back in his chair, thought a moment, then nodded. "O.K., when I go back to playing tennis, I'll work on it."

I shook my head. "You're going to have to start working on that a lot sooner than when you walk out on the tennis court. Starting today you're going to have to take up a new sport that's going to be very tough on you."

"What?" he asked suspiciously.

"Listening."

"What?"

"Yes, just listening, without thinking about the million problems in your business. Listening to your wife, your children, your friends, people who mean something to you, acquaintances, anyone who's talking to you, even if he's a doctor. Just hear what they're saying and think of what they're saying, even if it won't help you in business or winning a tennis tournament, just—"

". . . pay attention!" He said brightly, "See, I listened to everything you were saying without thinking of another thing."

"And another thing—"

"I know. Stop finishing people's sentences for them."

I had to laugh.

"O.K.," I said. "Let's try something." He lifted his chin challengingly. "Type A's are notorious for not being able to listen to long rambling statements. Well, this one is going to be long and I can't guarantee that I won't ramble, but I want you to bear with me for a moment. The point of it all is at the end."

Actually, I wasn't going to test his attention span so

much as make the point of what I had to say to sink in. He settled back in his chair, looking alert.

"The job of your arteries," I said, "is to supply oxygen and food to the cells in your body. The branch arteries work on a sort of buddy system. If a branch artery fails, another artery nearby can take over while still supplying its own cells. It does a double job. Now, that's how it works in the body and that's also the way it works in the heart. If a coronary artery gets stopped up, there is an interconnecting system from the other coronary arteries which will help to take over. But this system takes time to develop, and frequently, at the beginning of the coronary, there's not enough time. The piece of muscle tissue that the artery was supplying is in immediate trouble, and that's one of the reasons why heart attacks are almost always synonymous with emergencies."

Frank was listening so intently he was practically mouthing my words after I said them. But he couldn't resist interrupting to ask, "What do you mean by interconnecting system?"

"Just listen, don't talk!" I said. "Now, if the heart can survive the first shock of that tissue dying, then another, really miraculous process begins: the coronary arteries near the injury start enlarging and filling with more blood and, even more important, new branch vessels and connections actually begin growing in order to bring blood to the area. This improvised blood supply is called collateral circulation. You follow me so far?"

"Oh, sure. I read all that. I mean—" he waved toward the books, "I skimmed all that. But," he added triumphantly, "I listened to you with both ears and what's in between."

"Good. Now here's my point. If your heart can perform

such a miracle of regeneration as collateral circulation for you, then you can certainly make the effort to convert from a Type A to a Type B for your heart, right?"

"O.K.," Frank nodded firmly. "Good as done. From now on, I'm going to be a Type B."

"I wish it were as easy as that," I said, "but it isn't."

"I don't see what's so difficult!" Frank snapped. "If I make up my mind to, I can change from a Type A to a B faster than—" He stopped uncertainly. "Faster than what?" he muttered to himself. "What the hell am I competing against?" He fell silent.

I stood up.

"For your first day," I said, "don't you think you've been out of bed long enough?"

"Yeah." He was thinking, but it wasn't polyphasic thinking, because he was hardly paying attention to me.

"I'll help you back in."

"O.K."

When he was lying in bed he said, "It might be a little tough to change the habits and thinking of a lifetime."

"It won't be easy, but I'd say you've got a lot of reasons for the incentive."

"Guess so. I've just come through a coronary. So I'll always know there's one thing a lot tougher than changing thinking and habits—another coronary. I'll figure a way to dump the Type A thinking."

"I hope so."

"You'll see. This time I'm not just sounding off. I mean it."

Now was the time, I thought, to get a commitment.

"Would you like to prove it," I said, "right now?"

He looked at me warily. "How?"

I held out my hand. "Let me have your wristwatch. I'll give it to your wife next time I see her and she'll put it away."

"I don't get it."

"Well, a Type A lives by the clock. A Type B doesn't. Certainly not while he's in a hospital, so why do you need a watch here?"

Frank looked at my hand a moment, then unstrapped the watch.

"Atta boy."

"Wait a minute." He plucked a small, leather-covered traveling clock off his night table, snapped it shut and handed it to me also.

"By God, Frank, you realize this means ten extra brownie points?"

He sighed, shaking his head. "You know how many years I've been waking up and hearing that ticking?"

"From now on, you can wake up and listen to your heart ticking," I told him, "and think how much longer you'll be listening to it now that you're going to be a Type B." I checked my own watch. "And while you're still in the hospital, you can plan your new life. It'll be a long while till you have this much time on your hands with no distractions. You ought to come up with some dandy ideas."

"Ideas for what?"

"Hobbies, diversions, avocations, pastimes, arts, crafts. You name it."

"How about you naming it?"

"Uh-uh. When it comes to laying out your second life, you're your own doctor. After all, you've got to live it. Just find hobbies and pastimes you can enjoy for their own sake without worrying about profit and loss. Think about it."

"Maybe that'll be my pastime."

"What?"

"Thinking about hobbies." He grinned.

"Sounds relaxing." I turned to go.

"Can't we talk about it some more?"

"What's the rush? After all, you've got another week here."

Frank opened his mouth then closed it, put his hands behind his head and lay back on his pillow. "Well, you're the doctor," he sighed.

I grinned. "I was wondering how long before you would come right out and admit it."

6. How to Succeed with Heart Failure

Jenny Rosen was my oldest patient—not in years of age (though she was eighty-one) but in years I'd known her in my practice. She had been coming to the office regularly for checkups and treatment since my first week in practice, fresh out of residency.

When she first came to see me with palpitations her husband would close his kosher butcher shop in order to accompany her to my office, then take her home. Now the chore was done by her son, who once a month took time off from his job as manager of a supermarket to drop his widowed mother off. He would return an hour later to drive her back to her tiny apartment, which was a block away from his own.

On this particular visit when I asked the plump, motherly little woman how she was, she said, "Oh, *this* week I feel fine, Dr. Karpman."

The slight emphasis was of course for my benefit. "What do you mean '*this* week,' Jenny?"

She took price in the fact that I called her by her first name. At the same time she rarely addressed me without using both my medical title and last name.

She heaved a sigh. "Oh, last week, Dr. Karpman, I felt just terrible."

I assumed a concerned expression, which I knew she always found to be reassuring. "Why didn't you phone me then?"

"Oh, no, Dr. Karpman," she replied, looking appalled, "I didn't want to worry you."

It's that sort of utterance from a patient like Jenny Rosen that can make a doctor's day.

"But that's what I'm here for, Jenny. Now, what happened last week?"

"All of a sudden I woke up in the middle of the night and I couldn't breathe."

"How do you mean?"

"Like this, Dr. Karpman." She demonstrated with a series of short, shallow breaths.

"I see. Did that happen before you went to bed or afterwards?"

"After I was in bed. I fluffed up my pillow and went to sleep and an hour or two later it happened."

"Do you sleep on only one pillow, Jenny? You used to sleep on two. Remember, you told me you slept better with two."

"Three," she corrected, "but lately my arthritis feels better if I lay flatter in bed, so for the past couple of months I've been sleeping with only one pillow. I meant to tell you, Dr. Karpman, but I've been so busy with cooking and what not, I just forgot." She sighed, smoothing her flowered print dress over her lap with her small, capable hands.

"O.K., Jenny, so you fluffed up your pillow and went to sleep, and an hour or two later you couldn't breathe. What did you do then?"

"I sat up in bed and I felt a little better, so I thought it's going away and I laid down and it got worse again. I got so frightened, Dr. Karpman. I thought, oh, my God, this is the end! It's not so much me, Doctor. I'm no spring chicken, I'm already seventy-eight"—she pared off three years without a blush—"my daughters are settled with good husbands and lovely children, but what will happen to poor David?"

Poor David was Jenny's son, then fifty-one.

"After it got worse, Jenny, what did you do?"

"I got up and opened the window wide—where I got the strength I'll never know—and breathed in and out like this." She took some deep breaths. "Then I waited till I *really* felt better."

"Did you feel bad when you laid down again?"

"No, because I didn't lay down this time, I was so nervous. I sat up in an armchair and dozed off and on during the night."

"Jenny, did you notice whether or not your ankles have been swelling recently?"

"Well, in fact they were swollen that night almost up to my knees. Of course, they're always swollen a little after I've been on my feet all day. Yes, come to think of it, they have been more swollen lately."

"You were on your feet all day before you had that attack of breathlessness?"

"How can you not be on your feet all day when you

make a six course dinner? No, seven. Fruit compote, chopped herring, matzoball soup, fricassee—"

"How many were there for dinner?"

"Well, my daughter from San Diego, my son-in-law, the four children, my oldest granddaughter's boyfriend, a lovely boy who's going to be a chiropodist, my David—that's eight."

"And you."

"I never sit down at the table. I'm too busy running back and forth . . ."

"Nobody helped you?"

"Who needs help? It's a small kitchen and I don't like anyone helping me," she said proudly, "not even with the dishes. I say to them, 'What do you think I am? An old lady?' "

"What did you eat for dinner, Jenny?"

"Who has time to eat? I was so busy. I did have some chicken soup, and I tasted the pot roast with the carrots and the potato kugel everybody said was delicious, only I thought it wasn't salted enough."

"You salt your food a lot?"

"Well, you got to bring out the taste."

"One more question, Jenny." This was the one that invariably turned her cheeks pink. "Do you still go to the bathroom to empty your bladder in the middle of the night?"

The blush came on schedule. "Not always," she answered, without looking at me.

"Did you go to the bathroom the night you had trouble with your breathing?"

She studied the framed diplomas on the wall as she shook her head.

"Why not?"

She coughed, took a small handkerchief out of her birds-nest purse, delicately patted her mouth with it, and put it back. Her cheeks were still pink. "I didn't feel like it till morning."

"O.K., Jenny," I said, getting up. "Let's go and take a look at you."

We went into the examining room and I carefully checked her for any evidence of fluid retention in the lungs, liver, and legs. Twenty minutes later we were back in my office. I explained to Jenny what had happened.

"Jenny, it was that seven-course family dinner you cooked and served and cleaned up after that did it."

"But Dr. Karpman, what did I eat? Nothing! Maybe a little soup . . ."

"It wasn't just the eating, it was also all that work. You overtired yourself and you had an attack of paroxysmal nocturnal dyspnea. That means shortness of breath that comes in spurts when you're in bed at night and that can lead to pulmonary edema."

"Pul-monary e-dema," she repeated carefully. I could almost hear her saying it importantly to the other senior citizens sunning themselves in the central court of the old apartment building where she lived. *My doctor says I've got pulmonary edema.*

"I've got a neighbor, Mrs. Sachs," Jenny sniffed, "a regular know-it-all. You know what she had the nerve to tell me I had that night? A heart failure!"

"She was right, Jenny."

"Heart failure!" She looked stricken. "But you just said . . . Heart failure! Oh, my God!"

"Now wait, Jenny, heart *failure* isn't a heart *attack.* It merely means that sometimes when you overexert yourself, your heart fails to pump enough blood to keep up with your effort, and the body gives up trying for a minute. Have you ever seen a track meet where athletes run against each other?"

"Where a man shoots a gun in the air and everybody runs in—what looks like underwear? Yes, sometimes David watches it on my television when he comes over."

"Well, if you watch those runners, you'll see at the end of the race sometimes one of them will collapse."

"Yes, but they just faint. They don't die, do they, Dr. Karpman?" She looked at me anxiously.

"Oh, no. Let me explain. When the athlete is running, his heart pumps faster and faster to supply oxygen in order to create the energy he needs for running faster. Finally at the finish line, he makes a big demand on the heart for a final burst of energy. If it's too big a demand, the heart can't supply enough and the body just quits. The runner collapses. With the body not overexerting itself, its need for extra energy drops. The heart keeps pumping, but slower, and the fresh oxygen supplies new energy that brings the runner out of his collapse. That's what heart failure is. The heart, because of overwork, *fails* to give enough energy to the body when the body needs it."

Jenny was wide-eyed. "But, Dr. Karpman, I wasn't running; I didn't faint during the dinner. I kissed everyone goodnight, cleaned up the kitchen and went to bed, and all of a sudden in the middle of the night I can't breathe." She looked at me reproachfully. "What kind of stories are you making up, Doctor?"

"Stories? I don't follow you."

"First you tell me it's pul-monary something, then when I tell you Mrs. Sachs said it was heart failure, you admit it was heart failure. You can tell me the truth, Dr. Karpman," she said, smiling bravely.

"I *am* telling you the truth. Paroxysmal nocturnal dyspnea is a symptom of heart failure. It means that it's hard to breathe because of fluid in the lungs. You remember I once explained to you that the heart consists of two pumps? The left one pumps the blood all the way through the body and back to the right pump. The right pump sends it through the lungs to the left pump, which sends it back again through the body to the right pump."

Jenny nodded impatiently. "You explained all that."

"All right, sometimes for one reason or another—overexertion, anxiety, extra demands—one of the pumps tires or weakens and slows down. The other pump meanwhile is still pumping fairly normally. That's what happened to you that night of your heart failure. Your right pump was relatively O.K. That's the one that sends the blood through the lungs to the left pump. But your left pump wasn't working so good. It wasn't pumping the blood through the body as fast as it was receiving it from the lungs. So fluid was backing up in your lungs."

"Doctor, could you maybe say it again more slowly?"

"It's like having the faucets in the bathtub open full force, pouring water into the tub. The drain is open, but it's too small to empty the water as fast as it's coming in. What would happen?"

"I know what would happen! It once happened. I opened the drain and I was letting fresh water in to clean out the bathtub, and somebody called me on the telephone and when I got back the water had overflowed, even with the drain open. You should have heard my landlord—"

"Right, the faucet flow was too strong for the drain to keep up with, so the water kept piling up in the tub till it overflowed. Same with your heart. The right pump was delivering blood through the lungs to your left pump. The left pump couldn't pump it out fast enough, so the blood started to back up into the lungs. As the lungs filled up with blood, you found it harder and harder to breathe."

"So that's what happened!"

"That's not the whole story. While your left pump was weakening, less blood was going through your body. A lot of your blood circulates through the kidneys. When less blood is going through the kidneys, the kidneys don't work as well. They send less fluid to the bladder. And because of that, the bladder takes a long time to fill up. That's why you didn't feel like going to the bathroom that night."

"I see," Jenny nodded politely, ever the fastidious lady.

"Now you have excess water in your bloodstream and it has to go somewhere, and where does it go? Right down to your feet and legs. That's why when I suspect heart failure I look for swollen ankles."

"So that's why they were so swelled up so much extra this whole week!"

"Yes. I could have given you something to get rid of the swelling and to strengthen your heart. Why didn't you phone me?"

"What is this fluid that goes down to my ankles that you keep talking about?" Jenny asked, parrying my question with a question. "Isn't it blood?"

I shook my head. "It's the water part of the blood. Like the water that comes out of a blister when it breaks."

"Why does it go down to the ankles?"

"Gravity makes the fluid sink down to your ankles. But at night, when you're lying flat in bed, the gravity pulls the excess fluid into your lungs instead of your feet, and it causes congestion. That's why you felt better when you sat up in bed that night. The fluid drained down, the pressure went off your lungs, and you could breathe easier."

"And when I went back to bed again, my lungs got congested and I felt worse. What happens when it's the other side of the heart that doesn't work so good, Doctor?"

"You mean when the right pump that pumps blood into the lungs weakens? Well, the blood starts backing up behind the lungs and now not only the ankles swell, but the entire lower half of the body can swell. When tissues are filled with fluid, that's called edema. It used to be called dropsy."

"Dropsy! Of course!" Jenny's face lit up with recognition. "Why didn't you say so in the first place? My uncle and two aunts had it in my village in Russia when I was a young girl. They used to get swollen up like balloons from the waist down."

"All that fluid in their tissues. Sometimes when we get the heart to beat normally, a person can start urinating excess fluid."—Jenny looked at her hands discretely—"and he can lose as much as thirty or forty pounds, sometimes even more."

"But my heart is back to normal, isn't it, Dr. Karpman?" she asked anxiously.

"Not yet, but it's better than it was. I'm afraid that, for the time being, you're going to have to give up seven-course dinners for eight people." She sighed. "And you'll have to cut down on salt."

"Salt?" She looked pained. "How can you cut down on salt?"

"Salt is what keeps water in the body. After you've eaten something salty, you tend to take in and to keep more liquid in your system."

"That's true," she interjected sagely. "After pastrami for dinner, I could drink tea all night."

"And if your heart isn't working too well, your kidneys retain liquid and then you get swelling."

"But, Dr. Karpman, I got a friend who takes something to get the salt out of her system."

"A diuretic."

"That's just what she calls it."

"Oh, we can always use that, but I'd prefer to try more natural methods if we can. Just avoid salt and use salt substitutes.

"You mean it was the salt that did that to me?"

"Yes, both the salty food and all the work you did on that huge dinner that tipped you into heart failure. Your heart works fine for regular daily routines, Jenny, but don't push it too hard or you'll be in trouble."

Jenny shook her head, bewildered. "I don't understand. I've made dinners for fifteen, maybe twenty people when both daughters visit, and it didn't bother me then."

"Like you said, Jenny, we're not spring chickens anymore."

"You mean I'm an old lady, Dr. Karpman," she sighed.

"Jenny, you don't look a day over sixty-five."

She looked at me sadly. "I look that old?"

"A young sixty-five. But you've still got to watch yourself. And the first thing I'd want you to watch is your weight."

"You always want me to lose weight, Dr. Karpman. I lost three pounds from the beginning of this year, didn't I?"

"Now I want you to lose twenty more."

"Twenty pounds!"

"I want to get you down to what we call your dry weight."

She looked at me reproachfully. "You make me feel like a baby in diapers."

"Jenny, you've got too much water in your tissues. That's water weight. Besides you've got a little too much flesh weight. The less weight you carry around of any kind, the less chance of your waking up in the middle of the night and trying to catch your breath."

"But, Doctor, I promise I won't make any more big dinners or do all that going back and forth between kitchen and dining room!"

"Jenny, it's not only all the trips back and forth but also the extra weight you're carrying. That's weakening the heart pump. Your heart has to nourish all that fat on your body"—her face colored—"and when you're overweight, it has to work harder to nourish all that extra blubber. Even after we get the extra water out, you're going to have to slim down."

She winced and lifted her chin higher to make her neck appear less plump.

"Heart patients should be close to ideal body weight. Now, I want you to get your weight down twenty pounds, and I want you to get in the habit of weighing yourself every morning before breakfast. If you suddenly gain three or four pounds, you're to call me—I mean it—because you might be keeping water in your system and I'll have to give you some medication to get rid of it. We don't want to have another spell of heart failure on our hands."

"I'll call, I'll call," she said wearily.

"Just remember, anyone who's overweight is putting extra burdens on their heart. It's like a small car that's overloaded going up hill. It can break down."

Jenny sighed. "That's how it is with old people."

I shook my head. "With anybody. Any age. The moving around isn't what's bad for you. Being active is good for your heart. It keeps it in condition. But being heavy works against it. Smoking also works against it."

"I don't smoke."

I suppressed a smile. I could just imagine little, round Jenny Rosen with a cigarette in her mouth.

"And I'm proud of you for it. Now, Jenny, I'm going to give you a diet to follow. It cuts down on calories and on cholesterol."

I took some typed sheets out of my desk and handed them to her She took them carefully.

"Can I have another copy for my son, David?"

"Certainly." I gave her another set.

"Thank you, Dr. Karpman. Now, would you do me just one more favor, Doctor?"

"What's that?"

"Give David the same lecture about the heart you gave me? If you knew how he needs it!"

"Certainly. Tell him to call in any time for an appointment."

"He doesn't have to call, Doctor. He's out in the waiting room right now."

I was surprised to hear that. Usually, once Jenny's consultation was over, she would return to the waiting room and sit there patiently until her son showed up to take her home. As though reading my thoughts, Jenny said, "I asked him to wait for me this time. After what happened to me last week, I thought, who knows? Maybe I'll have to be rushed to a hospital, God forbid. So as long as he's here outside, maybe he could drop in for a second. Maybe you could squeeze him in on the end of my time." She smiled ingratiatingly. I couldn't help admiring how beautifully she had worked her subterfuge.

I could understand her concern when he came into my office. His father had proudly introduced him to me many years ago and he had been a nervous, lean young man. In the fifteen years since, however, he had gained a great deal of weight. But he had the alert, courteous manner of a good supermarket manager. After we greeted each other and shook hands, I said, "I was talking to your mother about controlling her weight. I can see that working around food must have its temptations, too."

He shrugged, "Oh, I can take it off any time I want."

"I'd say now is a good time, Dave."

I talked about the importance of losing weight, of a fat-controlled, low cholesterol diet, of regular exercise. He kept nodding attentively. When I handed him the diet sheets, he thanked me and carefully put them in his pocket. But the attentiveness seemed only skin deep, no doubt fostered by years of listening to housewives' complaints.

"The point I'm trying to make, Dave, is that if you lose weight, if you exercise, if you quit smoking, you're doing something to *prevent* a coronary and that's a whole lot better than *having* to do it after the coronary, right?"

"Absolutely, Doctor," he said. "You're one hundred percent right." Jenny beamed. Without thinking, David dipped into the pocket behind the MANAGER badge and pulled out a cigarette.

"Is that how you're proving it?" I asked as he struck a match.

"Is that how I'm proving what?" started David absently— then suddenly realizing, he fanned out the match, red-faced.

"Why don't you come in next week and we can discuss a program for you. My secretary will put you down . . ."

"I don't know about next week," David said, holding the unlit cigarette uncertainly. "We've got a big anniversary sale on and—"

"Listen to the doctor, David," Jenny said. "For your mother's sake."

"I *am* listening, Ma," he said with the irritation of a man who had been listening to his mother's admonitions for fifty-one years. "But I've got my hands full running the store and I wouldn't even know where to *begin* to find the time to start remodeling myself." He looked at his watch. "Are you finished up here, Ma? I've got to get back to work."

"Just a minute more," I told him. I cautioned his mother about not overexerting herself and about losing weight, and wrote out a prescription for a hundred digitalis pills. "If you ever get that hard-to-breathe feeling again, Jenny, sit up in a chair, breathe deeply, and then phone me."

Jenny took the prescription and looked at it with hostility. She didn't like to take pills.

"What kind of pill is it." she asked suspiciously.

"It's called digitalis and it strengthens the beat of your heart. It helps to prevent the fluid from backing up into your lungs. It was discovered two hundred years ago. An old lady in Shropshire, England, brewed a home-made tea that greatly benefited local people with dropsy. A physician, Dr. William Withering, heard about it and discovered that the tea was made from the dried leaves of a flowering plant called the foxglove. Those leaves contained digitalis, which can be a life-saver during heart failure. So you might say that old lady from Shropshire discovered a miracle drug."

Her face cleared. "A miracle drug I'll take anyday."

"Now Jenny, take one a day, every day. And don't run out of them."

As they started to leave, I suddenly recalled a passion that Dave had had many years ago. "If I remember, Dave," I said casually, "you used to be crazy about sports cars."

His eyes lit up. "Yep. Still am. Right now I drive a Jaguar 1100."

"The new one?" I asked.

He nodded proudly.

"Well! I understand they come not only with tools and instruction book but even a pair of coveralls so you can do your own repair work."

"Oh, yes. In fact, it's one of the things that sold me on the car."

I snapped the trap.

"Isn't it amazing, how much time and effort people spend keeping their cars in shape, but when it comes to keeping their heart in shape, they can't seem to get around to it."

David stopped grinning. "I find fooling around with cars relaxing," he said smoothly, "and that's good for the heart, isn't it?" He looked at his watch again. "Well, Ma, got to get back."

"Why don't you make an appointment with me for the week after your anniversary sale?" I called after him amiably.

"I'll try," he mumbled as he went out. "Nice to have seen you again, Doc."

"I don't think he liked what you said about his automobile," Jenny whispered to me fearfully as she trailed after him.

"That's fine, Jenny. Maybe it'll make him think."

I phoned Jenny two weeks later to find out how she was doing on her diet. She was more concerned in telling me about her son, and I was interested because he had made no attempt to make an appointment with me.

"Day and night, Dr. Karpman, I keep asking him when is he going to stop smoking and go on the diet and start exercising and go see you, and all he says is 'Soon, soon, stop nagging me.' I don't know what I'm going to do with him."

"Keep nagging. Now, let me ask you—are you following the diet?"

"Oh, yes."

"Are you losing weight?"

"Well—yes."

"Good."

"The first couple days, I lost all the extra water, no more swelling."

"And then?"

"Then no more."

"All right, Jenny, what's wrong?"

"Nothing's wrong, Dr. Karpman! I'm following the diet."

"Are you following it *exactly?*"

"Exactly! I swear on my late husband's grave, exactly! Except for a few changes."

"What changes?"

"Well, it says on your diet two strips of bacon a week, but I don't eat bacon. So I'm using chopped liver."

"Anything else?"

"It says Melba toast. I never liked Melba toast and it gets into my bridge."

"Than substitute matzoh."

"Matzoh! I never thought of that, Doctor."

"What did you substitute?"

"Bagel."

"Jenny, bagel is just as fattening as bread, maybe more."

"But I toasted it."

"Toasting doesn't burn off the calories."

"It doesn't?"

"Jenny, listen, no more bagels. Matzoh. No more chopped liver or chopped herring, O.K.? And when you come here for your next checkup we'll go through your diet and figure out substitutions for any of the foods on the diet that you don't usually eat."

"A good kosher diet is all I ask, Doctor."

"Fine. I'm also going to send you a refill on your prescription for diuretic pills."

"What?"

"The water pills. You should be taking one a day."

"Oh, Doctor, why do I have to take those? Mrs. Manhoff, she takes them to get the salt out of her system. But I've already given up on salt. I use a salt substitute. So I stopped the water pills."

"Jenny, never stop anything without asking me. Now, keep taking those water pills. You should take one every morning. And in an emergency, like if you're out of breath as you were that night, take one or two extra. O.K.?"

She sighed windily. "Yes, Dr. Karpman."

"Take it with a glass of orange juice."

"But orange juice has got fluid in it!" She sounded like a child catching a parent in error.

"It also has a lot of potassium in it, and potassium is needed in your system. When you're taking a diuretic, it sometimes can make the kidneys get rid of too much potassium in the urine and you therefore have to replace it."

"Yes, Doctor."

"I'll mail out the prescription right now, and when you get it, go right to the drugstore."

"There's a drugstore in David's market."

"Wonderful. I'll see you in a month."

A month hence would have been her regular checkup appointment, but I saw her a week earlier than that. There was an urgent call on my message service at three o'clock in the morning. Phone Jenny Rosen, emergency. Her son answered, his voice near hysteria. "She's trying to breathe,

Doctor, she's gasping. She could barely phone me to come over!"

It sounded like acute heart failure, pulmonary edema.

"Give her one of those water pills immediately!"

Diuretics are the most important agents for getting rid of fluids congesting the lungs in such a situation. They are also a simple way to get effective therapy started until other forms can be made available.

"She . . . she doesn't have any, Doctor."

I was stunned. "Why not?"

"She used them all up."

"Didn't she get the prescription refilled?"

"She asked me . . ." His voice faltered, "I hadn't gotten around to it yet. I was so busy . . ."

I could sense how choked up with guilt he was. Between his store and his sports car, he had been too occupied to get something that turned out to be crucial to his mother's health.

"Dave, I'm going to phone the Fire Department for a rescue squad to bring her some oxygen. Dave, do you hear me? *Dave!*"

"Sorry, Doctor, I was trying to get her to lie down but she fights me."

"*Don't* try to get her to lie down. Much better for her to sit up."

"Oh, my God, Doctor!"

"What is it, Dave. DAVE!!"

"Her lips are turning blue! It's like she's drowning!"

It was now unquestionable that Jenny Rosen was having an attack of acute left heart failure. The left ventricle, which pumps the blood out of the lungs and through the body, had weakened to the point where it could only pump a fraction of the blood coming to it from the lungs. Dave's panicky statement was accurate: the blood backing up in the lungs was literally drowning Jenny.

"What can I do, Doctor?!"

"Dave, a fire rescue squad will be there in a matter of minutes."

"But she might be *dead* by then!"

"She won't be—"

"SHE WILL!! Please, Doctor, tell me what to do! Please!!"

There *was* one thing he could do. Curiously, pulmonary edema is the one disorder for which "bleeding," the medieval panacia for *all* ailments, was genuinely effective. During acute left heart failure the lungs fill with a great volume of blood, and the medieval physicians, without really knowing what they were doing, helped victims of this by opening a vein and letting the patient bleed. As has been said, "it was a case of a stopped clock being right twice a day—the doctors helped a patient purely by accident."

I was not about to recommend bleeding, and indeed I would rarely recommend the technique I was about to tell Dave. But I now had two patients to contend with—one the victim of acute heart failure, the other the victim of acute guilt.

"O.K., Dave, here's what to do. Stand by the phone and I'll call you back in thirty seconds."

"Hurry!"

I hung up, called the Fire Rescue Squad and an ambulance, and dialed Dave back.

"Doctor, she's the same! *I've got to do something!*"

"All right, listen carefully. Do you know what a tourniquet is?"

"Sure. I was a Boy Scout."

"Good. O.K., first make sure she's sitting up as high as possible. Then put a tourniquet around each of your mother's arms to stop the circulation. Put them as high and close to the shoulders as you can. You know, around the armpits. Use ropes, string, handkerchiefs, socks, stockings, anything."

"All right."

"Then do the same thing around her thighs. As close to the body as possible."

"I can't do that."

"Why not?"

"She'd be so embarrassed."

"All right, then," I said, relieved, "just wait for the rescue squad." I would just as soon he not do anything.

"No, no, I'll do it! Please, Doctor!"

"Very well. Tighten three of the four tourniquets until you can barely feel a pulse, O.K.? In about five to ten minutes, loosen one of the tourniquets, tighten the one that was left off before, then rotate them every ten minutes. Keep doing it until the ambulance gets there, got that?"

"Right."

I hung up. The tourniquets would almost shut off the veins, damming up the blood in the extremities and thereby decreasing the flow of blood back to the right heart. The left heart would go right on pumping the blood out of the lungs, gradually alleviating the congestion in them. No matter how tightly Dave put the tourniquets on, there was little danger of hurting the tissues in Jenny's arms and legs, unless the tourniquets were left in place without being loosened for more than thirty minutes.

An hour later, in the hospital, propped up in bed with the pink back in her cheeks and her breathing normal, Jenny was both excited and embarrassed. "Wasn't my David something?" she said proudly. "The firemen said they'd never seen a what-you-call-it, a tourniquet, made from a venetian blind cord."

She then sheepishly recounted her previous evening. "I had the ladies from my canasta club over and I made a few refreshments. Nothing special, just some sponge cake and blintzes—everyone says I make better blintzes than in the store—and apple and prune strudel and a honey cake and fruit compote and—"

"And how many ladies came from the canasta club?"

"They all came. Why should anyone stay home?"

"How many were there?"

"Sixteen, including Mrs. Katz's sister, who—"

"Sixteen! And all that cooking! After I *told* you how overexertion could bring on heart failure. Jenny, I am really ashamed of you!"

"But I kept to my diet," she said bravely. "I didn't eat one thing I shouldn't."

"That's fine, but still!"

"And I promise I won't overwork myself. No more. I think I learned my lesson."

"I hope so, Jenny, but I'm not taking any chances. Once you're out of the hospital, you'll have to come to my office every week until I'm sure the amounts of digitalis and of water pills you'll be taking are just right."

"When will I be out of the hospital?"

"In a few days. Isn't that good news?"

Jenny nodded. Then she said with a smile, "I just had even better news."

"What's that?"

She brought out a crushed pack of cigarettes from under the pillow.

"Jenny! Isn't it a little late in life to start . . . ?"

"No, no, they're David's. He was sitting in the ambulance

with me and I said to him, 'See, David, what can happen if you don't follow the doctor's advice?' So he takes out his cigarettes and crushes them in his hands and he says from now on he's going to stop smoking, go on a diet, and start exercising."

She smiled at me beautifully. "Dr. Karpman, it was the best heart failure a mother could ask for."

7. A Case of Icy Fingers

"I had lunch with Allen last week," Joan said. She sighed. "He's impossible."

Joan Seberling, forty-two, was a strikingly handsome woman—tall, brunette, superbly groomed, and with an elegance appropriate to her position as head of a successful Los Angeles modeling school. She had been a divorcee for seven years but was on amiable enough terms with her ex-husband, Allen, to lunch with him weekly. Now she was seated in my office, beginning her first visit with an elaborate apology.

"I casually mentioned that now and then the palms of my hands seem to sweat up, while my fingers get icy cold. I thought it was interesting, that was the only reason I mentioned it, but Allen immediately insisted I see a doctor. He's such an old lady. I told him it was ridiculous to see a doctor about a matter like that, but you know Allen."

I did indeed know Allen. Some years ago he had come to me about minor palpitations, and after successful treatment we had become casual friends. Now sixty-one, he wrote instruction manuals for office machinery and hovered about his ex-wife as much as she would let him. Though he talked about Joan a great deal, this was the first time I had met her. She sat with a model's perfect poise, back straight, hands resting carefully in her lap.

"So he went and made this appointment and he's been phoning me all week to make sure I would keep it. One offhand remark and he turns into a mother hen!"

Many people are only comfortable going to a doctor if they are pushed into it, and I therefore feel quite strongly that remarks made "offhandedly" to mother hens are often unconsciously designed to provoke them into doing just what Allen had done. She was playing down her symptoms, something women patients don't usually do during the first consultation—unless they are women with a career.

"Are those the only things that bother you?" I asked. "Icy fingers and sweaty palms? Is there anything else? Take your time and try to remember."

"Well, a little shortness of breath every so often, but it's nothing much."

"You've had trouble breathing?"

"Oh, that would be overdramatizing it, though technically I suppose you're right. Actually, all I have is just these occasional cold hands. Now, really, does that justify my coming down here and wasting your time?"

"Tell me, Mrs. Seberling—"

"Oh, please," she interrupted, "I never use that name in my work. I'm Joan Ellen in the office."

"Miss Ellen, Mrs. Ellen, or Ms. Ellen?"

She smiled. "Why don't we just call me Joan?"

"Fine. Joan, when you get icy hands, do your feet get cold at the same time?"

"Didn't I mention that? Yes they do."

"How often do you get these icy hands and feet?"

"Every so often."

"What does that mean? Every day?"

"Oh, no. It depends. I think the last time it happened was probably last week in Chicago."

"Were you there on business or vacation?"

"Vacation? In Chicago?" She raised her eyebrows. "No, Doctor, my school is part of a chain, and our company headquarters are in Chicago. I went there for a meeting with the president to discuss a change of curriculum. Now there's a real fussbudget! He wants you to check with him on everything from buying make-up kits to going to the john."

"Did your cold hands start before, during, or after your meeting?"

"Before. My palms were sweating so I was afraid to shake hands with him. You never know what he might think."

"When was the time before that? Do you remember?"

"Yes, it was the beginning of this month, when I spoke to a Woman's Advertising League Monday morning brunch. It turned out to be fun. We all let our hair down and let fly at Madison Avenue."

"Did you get the cold hands before your speech?"

"Yes."

"Would you say in general that you get those symptoms *before* important conferences or speeches?"

"Yes, I get them when I'm uptight. But once I start talking and I know I'm coming over all right, then it goes away. It's something like stage fright."

"How long has it been going on?"

"A year or so. Wouldn't you say it's a form of stage fright?"

"We'll know better after you've been examined."

She looked apprehensive. "Examined?"

"Oh, it's nothing unusual. Blood pressure readings. Blood and urine tests. Electrocardiograph. Chest x-ray."

"All that just because my hands and feet get cold before making a speech?"

"Chances are you're fine, but with symptoms like yours it's just sensible to have a complete examination. When was your last checkup?"

"I don't have them."

"O.K., then we'll check out your icy hands and give you a physical at the same time. Why don't you have yearly checkups?"

"I don't think I need them. I haven't had a sick day in years."

"Not even a headache or an eye strain?"

"Well, everybody has those, occasionally. I get over them in no time."

"Do you ever get fatigued? That is, really exhausted?"

"Why shouldn't I?" Joan replied defensively. "When you work like a horse sometimes you get terribly tired, but I'm never sick. Certainly not enough to see a doctor. I know a lot of people go to one regularly, but for me to do that, well . . ." A graceful shrug indicated what a preposterous idea she thought that was.

"Do you go to a hairdresser regularly? To a gym? To a beauty salon?"

She smiled. "But of course. I go to beauty salons and hairdressers regularly and I work out in a gym three times a week. But that's different. As director of a modeling school, my appearance is vital to my job."

"Do you go regularly to a dentist?"

"Certainly, but for the same reason. My teeth are a very important part of my appearance."

"If you didn't go to him regularly," I said, "you wouldn't have those lovely teeth. Now isn't body health as vital to you as a lovely smile?"

Pointedly, she flashed her lovely smile. "You win. I'll make an appointment."

"You don't have to make an appointment. There's an examining room right down the hall."

Joan blinked. "How long will it take?"

"At the most an hour."

"An hour! I'll kill that Allen!" She turned a pendant watch to look at the time. "I'll have to call my office and postpone a staff meeting."

I turned my phone around on the desk. "Be my guest."

"Oh, thanks, but I wouldn't want to tie up your phone."

"You won't be. My secretary can always get to me through another line."

I had an ulterior motive in being gracious. I wanted to get a sampling of Joan's business personality. Other sides of a patient are sometimes at complete variance with the side presented to the doctor, and in Joan's case it could be significant. It was. Whereas Joan Seberling was, to me, voluble and charming, Joan Ellen was terse, tough, and humorless as she laid down to a secretary and a male subordinate exactly what was to be done at the staff meeting while she was away.

Significantly, she did not mention where she was or the reason for her delayed return. Obviously, she didn't want anyone at the school to know she was seeing a doctor. When she hung up, she confirmed this with a conspiratorial wink. "Our little secret, O.K.?"

Three days later she was back in my office for the report on her examination.

"The icy hands and feet," I told her, "plus the occasional breathlessness are symptoms of what is called functional vasospasms. It literally means 'mild contractions of the peripheral arteries.' The peripheral arteries are the ones in the fingers and the toes."

She looked at me, eyes wide. "It's not anything serious, is it?"

"Oh, no. At least not at present."

"What does *that* mean?"

"At present it's a very minor matter. As you may know, your main artery leaving the heart, the aorta, is like a tree trunk with smaller arteries branching out from it and still smaller arteries branching out from them. The next-to-smallest twigs, actually microscopic, are called arterioles. Now, when you are faced with a particular stressful situation, the arterioles tend to constrict. And the heart then has to pump harder to push blood through them."

"Is that why my heart was beating fast? Trying to pump blood through those shrunken little pipes?"

I smiled at the aptness of her description. "Right. When the arterioles shrink, blood moves more slowly, the blood flow to your extremities is significantly reduced, and less oxygen is getting through to your tissues. That's why your hands and feet get cold."

"I don't get it."

"Well, blood is warm. Less blood to the fingers and toes means less heat to those fingers and toes. That's why when people are cold, they try to increase their circulation by rubbing themselves or exercising. The heat energy opens up the arterioles.

"I get the picture. So after I stop being tense, the little pipes stop shrinking, more blood goes through them, and my hands and feet start feeling warm again."

This was a bright lady.

"Exactly."

Joan gave me her gorgeous smile. "Well, it's just like I thought. It was hardly worth coming to see you. Wait till I see that mother hen Allen. By the way, what about my palms sweating?"

"Nothing really important. Most people with functional vasospasms have perspiring palms, some don't. Let's call it a quirk of the individual's nervous system."

"Well," said Joan, picking up her handbag and making motions to go. "As long as it's not important."

"What *is* important," I said, "is that vasospasms sometimes are the first warning that a person may be a candidate for hypertension."

Her calm was suddenly replaced by apprehension. "Isn't that like high blood pressure?"

"It's the same thing."

Her reaction was astonishing. She sprang to her feet, elegance gone. "Of all the goddamned . . . !"

"Hey, take it easy! I don't know why you're carrying on so. You're a very lucky woman!"

She stared at me in disbelief. "You tell me I've got high blood pressure and you say I'm *lucky?* I'm the only woman running a school in this chain. I've got an assistant, Brady, after my job. I've got a chairman of the board and president of the corporation, J.G., who only has to get word that I've got high blood pressure . . ."

"I said you were only a candidate."

"That won't matter to J.G. He'll tell the board, 'See what you get when you put in a woman director?' and I'll be out on my ass. Goddamn that Allen! If he hadn't phoned you . . ."

"Come on, Joan, all you're doing is getting your blood

pressure up. Now, in the first place, high blood pressure doesn't prevent anyone from doing their job . . ."

"Go tell that to Chicago! He didn't want a woman in the job to begin with, but I'm damn good, and the board knew it and they voted me in. All J.G. needs is one good excuse, and Brady is just panting to get something on me, the bastard!"

"How's he going to find out anything? Not from me, certainly."

"And I don't want Allen to know either. He's such a damned blabbermouth."

"My lips are sealed."

She smiled suddenly. "Look, I'm sorry about the outburst, but you don't know how I've been dreading getting something that would give them a chance to say, 'Put a woman in a man's job and she gets sick.' And you tell me I've got high blood pressure and then you tell me I'm a lucky woman . . ."

"But you *are* lucky and you don't *have* high blood pressure. You're lucky to find out now that you have a tendency toward developing it. Millions of people with high blood pressure don't even know they have it."

"And I wish I were one of them."

"You wish you didn't find out until you were on the road to kidney failure or congestive heart failure or stroke or coronary artery disease? That's the worst nonsense I've ever heard! Sit down and let me explain something."

She sat down and looked at me broodingly.

I picked up her medical report. "We took your blood pressure several times during your checkup. The average was 145 over 92."

"What does that mean?"

"Blood pressure is created by the contractions of the

heart muscle pumping blood through the blood vessels and by the resistance of the walls of the artery."

She looked at me dully, the look of someone getting over a shock; but she was listening, and that was important.

"Now the heart," I went on, "is not one but two pumps. The right one pumps blood through the lungs to pick up oxygen. Then the left one pumps the oxygenated blood through the arterial system of the body. When the left chamber contracts and squeezes blood into the arteries, that moment of left heart contraction is the point of maximum pressure. It's called the systolic pressure. Then when the chamber opens again to receive another load of blood, the pressure in that moment of slack is at minimum. That minimum pressure is called the diastolic pressure. Yours is 92. So your maximum and minimum pressure is expressed as 145 over 92. That's borderline high. The ideal for someone your age is 120 or 130 over 80."

"And that little bit extra means I've got high blood pressure?"

"I didn't say you had it, Joan."

"That I was a candidate for it?"

"There's other evidence. The cold hands and feet during anxious periods, the tension you feel. That's why I asked you if you had headaches or eye strain or ever felt extremely fatigued."

"You mean when you have headaches or eye strain or feel tired, you're on the way to high blood pressure?" The fusillade of questions indicated she had perked up a lot. There was a lot of bounce-back in this woman.

"Not necessarily. Only occasionally do cold hands and feet mean high blood pressure. But when you put them together, they start adding up." I looked at her medical coronary report. "Your mother's father died of a coronary occlusion and her mother died of kidney failure. You told me your mother has angina pectoris. Right there are three cases in which high blood pressure could have played a part."

"How?"

"Well, if the arterioles stay constricted, then the heart has to pump harder without letup. The arteries begin having too much pressure in them, and little breaks and rips appear on the inside walls, like a hose with too much water forced through it. Fatty deposits in the blood get caught in those tears, and soon atherosclerosis starts building up. The result may be angina pectoris or even a coronary, as happened with your grandfather. With your grandmother, athersclerosis in the kidneys may have produced the kidney failure . . ."

"All right, I get the picture. Once I told you about my grandparents and my mother and you took my blood pressure, you knew I was a-a . . ."

"Potential hypertension victim, yes. With the added factor of the cold hands and feet, the headaches . . ."

"If you knew it that soon," Joan interrupted indignantly, "why did you put me through that long physical exam?"

"For one thing, I was looking for everything I could that would either confirm or contradict my hunch. For instance, when I scanned the inside of your eye with that ophthalmoscope, I was examining the arterioles in the back of the eye. It's the only place in the body where we can actually see the arteries. People who have had high blood pressure for a long time have damaged arterioles from all the years of blood being pumped through them at high pressure. Your arterioles are still in excellent shape."

"Thank God for small favors."

"I also wanted to find out if you had what's known as secondary hypertension."

"What's that?"

"High blood pressure caused by some other ailment. It could be from a kidney disorder or a slight malfunction of the adrenal gland or even an abnormality of the aorta, the main artery of the body."

Joan blanched. Her bosom began to rise and fall. "Doctor," she murmured.

I hastened to add, "But your examination showed no signs of any of those. Matter of fact, if it had, it would have been possible to cure you, and one of the side benefits would have been the automatic clearing up of your tendency toward hypertension. However, secondary hypertension shows up in at the most ten percent of all high blood pressure cases."

"But I don't have it." There was relief in her voice.

"No, the kind of hypertension you have a tendency toward having is the most common kind. It shows up in ninety percent of the cases. It's called essential hypertension, or primary high blood pressure."

"What does that mean?"

I braced in anticipation of her shocked reaction. "It means we don't know what causes it."

Joan's lips parted. "Doctors don't know what *ninety* percent of high blood pressure is caused by?"

"Joan, there are many ailments we don't know the cause of but we know how to treat."

A small smile came to her lips. "That's like the story of the man who invented a cure for which there was no known disease."

I laughed. "Well, we do know the disease in this case, but

we don't exactly have a cure. What we do have are procedures and drugs for bringing down high blood pressure and keeping it down. Most important, we can prevent the complications like heart attacks, strokes, and kidney trouble."

"That's practically the same as a cure, isn't it?"

"Not exactly. You see, in each case of high blood pressure we have to experiment with different kinds of drugs in different combinations, and then the patient has to keep taking them to keep his blood pressure normal."

"How long?"

"Usually indefinitely."

She put on a woebegone face.

"So I'll have to take pills the rest of my life?"

"Hold on, Joan. You're not up to that. I told you you're a *candidate* for hypertension. You haven't been admitted to the club yet."

"What can I do to get blackballed?"

"For one thing, give up smoking. Cigarettes raise your blood pressure. You can also cut way down on your salt intake. You know how thirsty you get after eating anything salty? Salt in your system tends to make you take in more liquid and retain it in your tissues."

"At the school whenever any of the modeling students have weight problems we advise them to take diuretics to lose water weight."

"Doctors do too, on occasion, but I'd rather try doing things naturally before advising pills."

Joan took a deep breath and said briskly, "O.K. Cigarettes out, cut down on salt. Go on."

"Well, if you were overweight, I'd say diet. But you're obviously in, ah, very good shape."

She smiled, adept at accepting compliments. "It's always nice to be told that, especially by one's doctor."

"I'm sure you eat sensibly and go easy on cholesterol and all that."

"I'm always on a diet. It goes with the territory."

"Now there's one other thing you should do, and it's the toughest of all. Give up your tensions."

She looked at me grimly. "Are you saying I should give up high pressure? In other words, give up my job?"

"No, I mean give up your attitude. Get a low-pressure attitude toward a high-pressure job."

"Now, how am I supposed to do that?"

"You'll have to work on it. High-pressure lives, constant hostility, anxiety, emotional stress are great contributors to high blood pressure. If you can stop feeling such hostility and anxiety and fear in your work, you could possibly do more—"

"How can I?" Joan asked, "when I'm the only woman holding down a top job in a business where the men around me are trying to take it away from me *because* I'm a woman. Sure, I'm full of hostility and anxiety. Can you blame me?"

"You know that blacks in this country have a much higher incidence of high blood pressure than whites."

"I can see why. When you're a minority and you're always dealing with prejudice and hate and fear, I guess you're going to have higher blood pressure."

"Could be. You've got to get a better perspective on your job. You've got to start seeing it as only *part* of your life, not the whole thing. People who can leave their work when they leave the office generally—I said generally—don't have hypertension."

"Unfortunately, I don't seem to be one of them."

"Fortunately, you have time to change."

Joan sighed. "I suppose I ought to be thankful that Allen is such an old mother hen."

"I think you're right."

"On the other hand," she added almost venomously, "I wish he had minded his own business and not made me come to see you."

"Why not?"

She shrugged. "Well, I was feeling perfectly all right outside of those occasional anxiety reactions. So what was the big deal? As you yourself said, people go a long time without even knowing they have it."

"Ignorance is bliss, is that it?"

"Well, hell, knowing I'm on the edge of high blood pressure only boosts it higher. You've just given me added tension."

"Talk about female logic!" I exclaimed. And could have bitten my tongue.

"Why doctor," she said triumphantly "You're what they used to call a male chauvinist pig!"

"No, no. It was just that marvelous bit of reasoning you did made me forget myself."

"Appeal denied!"

By this time she was laughing. Easy, relaxing laughter—probably one of the healthiest drugs known.

"Seriously, though," I said, "wouldn't you prefer to go through the anxieties and troubles of readjustment now rather than be forced to do it the hard way by having a coronary?"

"I may sound a bit smug," Joan said, "but as I understand it, men are many times more susceptible to coronaries than women are—at least up to the time of menopause. I believe it's our estrogen that protects us from heart attacks."

"That was before women started coming out of the kitchen. But since they invaded the business world like you, they've been paying all the anxiety and tension penalties. These days, when it comes to coronaries, atherosclerosis, strokes, angina pectoris, women are closing the gap with men."

Joan shook her head ruefully. "We fight for equality with men and what do those bastards do? They hand us their coronaries. Is that what's called poetic justice?"

"And on top of it, you have the extra tension and anxiety of being discriminated against as a woman."

"Doctor, I hereby clear you of all charges of being a male chauvinist pig."

"Thank you. Now ease off on the tensions. Learn to enjoy life more."

"But I do enjoy life!"

"Then get a new, larger definition of life other than the rat race. Get a real social life. Hobbies, theater, music, vacation trips."

"I'll do it."

I wish she had. Both of us would.

8. Beating the Competition

The day after I talked with Frank about developing relaxing hobbies, I found him in an armchair in his room, sketching on a huge drawing pad. He was so intent that he didn't even notice me until he had finished drawing and turned to a new sheet. Then he waved his pencil.

"Hi, Doc." He didn't add the usual "How'm I doing?" Evidently he had given himself the seal of approval and had no need of mine.

"Morning, Frank."

"See," he said, "I'm Type B." The pencil resumed racing across the page.

"What are you drawing?"

"Girls. You said find a relaxing pastime, didn't you?" He sounded curiously defensive in spite of his heartiness.

Craning my neck I could see women's figures forming swiftly under his surprisingly skillful hands. He filled in a silhouette with neckline and pleats.

"That's a fashion layout, isn't it?"

He shrugged. "As long as I'm doodling, I figured I'd jot down some ideas. You know—just so it shouldn't be a total loss."

I noticed a fashion magazine on the table opened to a full page picture of a model in a low-cut jersey and pleated skirt. "Are you copying dresses?"

"Yep. And simplifying the designs. I'm cutting out all the gimmicks that make the original so expensive. Then we can turn out copies at twenty-five to fifty percent of the cost."

"You mean you're stealing the design?"

"Of course! Everybody in the cut-rate field does. When you sell garments at a big turnover for only pennies profit on each item, you gotta cut corners, and a designer's fee is the first corner to go. Everyone copies."

"But not as well as you, I'll bet." I watched his pencil move. "You're pretty good."

"Pretty good, hell! You're looking at one of the best fashion-magazine design lifters in the wholesale business. The Seventh Avenue Mafioso. You may be an expert in medicine, Doctor, but when it comes to this line of work—"

"Exactly. 'This line of work.' The day after you promise to turn into a Type B, I find you doing piecework in your hospital room. You can't go to work, so you bring your work here."

He stopped drawing and looked at me reproachfully. "Doctor, cross my heart, I find this very relaxing. I *enjoy* drawing, believe me."

"And it helps business. To quote a certain guy in soft goods: 'just so it shouldn't be a total loss.' "

"What's the matter with that?"

"Just this. Any time you're doing work, there's some tension quality in it, and tension and pressure is just what you should be trying to unlearn."

"Doc," his voice throbbed with sincerity, "believe me, I would enjoy this work just as much if it didn't bring me in a dime."

"I believe you. Now, let's prove it."

Frank groaned. "Every time you say 'Let's prove it,' I'm in trouble."

"On the contrary, I hope you're getting *out* of trouble. Now, I want you to prove you can perform this hobby of yours when it's bringing you nothing but aesthetic satisfaction."

"Look, what do I know from aesthetic satisfaction? All I am is a dress manufacturer . . ."

". . . who doesn't want to have a second coronary."

"All right. What do you want me to do?"

"Let me see you sketch something besides models in Paris outfits."

"But that's all I know how to draw!"

"How about drawing them without outfits?"

"You mean naked? My God, don't you doctors see enough of that?"

"I'm just trying to get you to branch out. I figured going from dressed models to undressed models would be an easy first step."

"And what comes after that?"

"Well, maybe you'll get interested in drawing for its own sake, in art. Then perhaps you'll start going to galleries . . ."

"How about porno films?"

"O.K., porno films, if that's what will teach you to relax and enjoy."

"Jesus, why can't I just keep copying these things?" His voice was plaintive. He finished another sketch and turned the page.

"Nobody says you can't. You're doing something you

enjoy that brings you profit. Fine. But that's no new pattern in your life. What would be new is learning to enjoy things for the sake of doing them."

I sat down opposite him. I wanted as much of his attention as I could get for what I had to say next. "The toughest thing a person can do in their middle years is to learn to grow. You have this talent for drawing. You're lucky. You can grow with that."

"Why can't I grow with tennis instead?"

"You'll go back to playing it, Frank, but it won't be for growing."

"Why not?" He grinned. "Frank Justin, tennis bum."

"I like the bum part. That's Type B. But your brand of tennis is competitive, and being competitive is one of the things you've got to learn to outgrow."

"You expect me to get to a point where I don't want to compete anymore?"

"I'd like you to get so you won't want to compete *all the time.* So you'll do things for the fun of it and find it rewarding."

"What am I supposed to find rewarding? Imitating bird calls?"

"If you enjoy it, sure. For you, rewarding should be anything that has nothing to do with profit or competition. Reading, taking courses, listening to music, bull sessions with your son, family picnics, photography, raising flowers, looking at sunsets, folk dancing, amateur acting—you name it. It's not so much a question of giving anything up. It's what you're going to add to your life. New interests can make you blossom . . ."

Frank held up the drawing he had been working on. "How's this for a blossom?"

He had filled the entire sheet with a drawing of a nude Amazon of remarkable proportions.

"I don't think you could get her into one of your dresses," I said, "but if I were a calendar company I'd give you a contract right now."

"How about being my salesman for twenty-five percent commission?"

"Will you stop trying to turn a buck, Frank, and just keep drawing?"

"Naked women?"

"Sure, if you enjoy it."

"Are you sure all this sex isn't dangerous for my heart?"

"As long as it's only on paper, we'll take the chance."

"Speaking of sex, Doc," he said, trying to sound offhand, "I've been reading this book"—he pulled a book off the night table, *Sex and Your Heart,* by Myron Benton—"and it says a lot of doctors are too inhibited to bring up the subject of sex to their patients. Are you one of them, Doctor?" He slyly emphasized the "Doctor."

"What do you think, Frank?" A doctor shouldn't duck any issue a patient is concerned about where it pertains to his heart.

"All right, then, when do I get my sex talk?"

I was certainly planning to give him a sex talk. But today wasn't the day. There were other things he had to know first. I moved my chair closer to his and leaned toward his ear. "O.K., Daddy," I said in a stage whisper. "What do you want to know?"

He laughed a little too hard. "Well, ah . . ." He was suddenly hesitant. "I'm still scheduled to go home next week, right?"

"Right."

He became silent, and his sketching movements became more rapid. He seemed to regret having raised the subject. I decided to help him out.

"You realize that once you get home, sex isn't your first priority."

"It isn't?" There was a note of relief. "Well, what is?"

"First, we have to get your diet and your regular exercise schedule running smoothly."

"We don't have to worry about the exercise. Once I can get back to tennis, I'll be in great shape."

"I said *regular* exercise, not just weekends."

"The way I play tennis, I make up for the other five days."

"I'm sure. Five days of sitting on your butt in an office, then two days of slamming around on a tennis court. That kind of stop-and-go exercise is hell on your heart, and would be even if you didn't have heart trouble. It's especially demanding when someone is a good player, and you are. A lot of standing around mixed with short bursts of action. You're going to need exercise of a more continuous, controlled nature for your heart. Anyway, you're not going to be able to play tennis for a while."

"How long is a while?"

"Frank, two weeks ago, the blood flow through one of your small coronary arteries was blocked. Result: the muscle tissue beyond that block was injured and a scar is forming. Developing a strong scar is a slow business, and while it's going on, the demands on the heart have to be very light. So, let's lay off planning your tennis comeback a while anyway."

"O.K., O.K. When do I start exercising?"

"You've started already."

I enjoyed Frank's look of surprise. "When?"

"You're in an armchair now, aren't you? Well, you had to get out of bed to get into it. And in a short while you're going to go back to bed."

"Yeah, I see. Of course the nurse helps me."

"It's still exercise. Also you've been shaving yourself. And your commode's been taken away, hasn't it?"

"That wasn't me. That was the night nurse's exercise."

"But since it's gone, you've been going to the bathroom. How many times?"

"Twice," Frank sighed. "I don't think they'll give Olympic medals for that."

"And before you leave next week, we're going to have you walking around the room at least twice a day."

"Well, it's no marathon, but it's something."

"The first day you're home, you should take it easy, mostly in bed, but then you can resume the routine you've had here for the past several days. You can get up to go to the bathroom and to the table for your meals. But after each meal I want you to rest for at least an hour. You can read or doze or whatever. You can sit in the living room and watch television whenever you feel up to it."

"Watching television sounds like great exercise."

"I'm just getting to the exercise. After you've been home a day or two, start walking around your room two or three times. Do it twice a day. Then increase the number of times you walk around the room or the house and the length of the walk until you're exercising for fifteen or twenty minutes."

"Taking my pulse all through this, huh?"

"Who told you that?"

"I read it."

"Well, your pulse, of course, is the best measure for determining whether you're pushing yourself too hard or too easy in your exercises. Some doctors don't like their patients to take their own pulse . . ."

"What are they afraid the patients are doing?" Frank asked. "Practicing medicine without a license?"

"No, it's just that some patients start feeling their pulse *all* the time. They get to be pulse freaks, so some doctors prefer that the patient's spouse handle it."

Frank looked disgusted. "Do I look like the kind of a guy who's going to join Pulse Feelers Anonymous?"

I smiled. "O.K., the easiest way to count your pulse is put a hand over your heart. But if you're wearing a heavy sweater or something, it might be easier to take it over the carotid arteries, which are on both sides of your neck. If you put either thumb on your chin, your fingers can easily feel the carotid artery in front of the strip of muscles running vertically in the neck."

"What about the wrist?"

"That's a good place. Take it on the thumb side of the wrist. Another place is inside the elbow toward the body side, or even in the groin."

"Not the groin, thanks," Frank grinned. "If anyone saw me, they might get the wrong idea."

"Very funny."

"Anyway, when do I take my pulse?"

"When you exercise. Take it resting and then take it *immediately* upon stopping exercise, because the rate slows very quickly after you stop exercising. Find the beat and count it for ten seconds. Then multiply by six to obtain the count for a full minute. Don't count for a whole minute or even for fifteen seconds, because the fall-off is too fast. At this stage, if your pulse goes over a hundred beats a minute, you're through for the day. It means you're pushing too hard so you rest."

"I'd think that a fast pulse means that your heart is getting exercise."

"If you found your heart rate to be very fast after a minimal degree of exercise and especially after having been at relative bed rest for two to three weeks in the hospital, chances are it means you're simply doing too much for your heart *at that time*. But after a period of gradually increasing exercise, it'll take longer for your heart rate to speed up. A trained athlete can walk rapidly for fifteen minutes or even thirty minutes around the room, and his heart rate might never go above fifty or sixty beats per minute. But non-athletes' hearts might speed up to one hundred beats per minute within a minute or two."

"You mean that athletes can have normal pulses of only fifty ticks a minute?"

"Oh, yes. An athlete with a heart muscle that has been exercised and developed to deliver a lot of blood with each pump can, when he's resting, have a heart rate of even less than fifty. Of course, his heartbeat can go way up if he's running the hundred-yard dash, but for a stroll around a room it should be only fifty or sixty. If at this stage you can do that same stroll at a heart rate of no more than ninety, I'll be happy. As your heart strengthens with regular exercise, the pumping will deliver more blood per beat and your heart rate won't go as high for the same amount of exercise."

"But if my pulse is too high, I don't get to do any exercise?"

"If your heartbeat gets too high after a minimal amount

of exercise, we'll have to scale down the exercise each day until your heart muscle tones up. I don't think we're going to have that kind of a problem with you since you've made such a good recovery. In any case, don't let your heart rate get over one hundred beats per minute for the present. O.K., now, after two weeks we'll check you over, and if everything's all right you'll start walking out of doors. Is the street you live on level or hilly?"

"It's level for four blocks, then it gets hilly on all sides. You know, woods, rocks, and things. I live in a canyon. Looks something like this."

With an economy of line he sketched his house and street on a sheet of paper. I noticed he couldn't resist putting in four faces staring out of the windows, obviously those of his wife and children.

"O.K., you'll start out walking a half-block twice a day, and after a month you ought to be doing eight or ten blocks."

Frank tapped his sketch. "But there are only four level blocks."

"I know. So you'll go back and forth until you've made up ten blocks. After the first month, I'll let you break out into the woods and rocks. Do your walking early mornings and late afternoons. And do it before breakfast and before supper or else wait at least an hour after meals before you start."

"Aye, aye, sir."

"And take someone with you for the first week or two."

"Why? Are you afraid I might drop dead in my tracks?"

"You could get tired unexpectedly those first few days, which means you could be better off with someone there." I tried to give his ego a boost. "Besides I'd like someone along to make sure you keep the walk *down* to what I prescribe. With you, it could turn into a cross-country hike into the next state."

He grinned. "I'll take Sheila along, and we'll talk about art and music and all that garbage so while I'm walking I'll be growing in my middle years."

I decided to ignore that.

"Two weeks from now, if everything's O.K., I'm going to let you go out evenings to a friend's home or to a movie . . ."

"With a companion, so I don't overdo it," he added dryly.

". . . and in about six weeks I'm going to drop your exercise program to three days a week, since by then, I expect, you'll be back to work part time—and a daily exercise program on top of working might be too taxing. Just the work itself will provide you with a certain amount of the exercise you'll need."

"How much is the part time?"

"You'll exercise and have breakfast, rest at least an hour, then get to the office at 10 o'clock or later. You'll work three or four hours, then quit for the day."

"Three or four hours! Hell, a forty-hour week used to be part time for me!"

"I'm glad you said 'used to be.' Now, about the exercise. The important thing is that it promote endurance and get the heart rate up within the target zone."

"What's the target zone?"

"It's when we have your heart beating fast enough during exercise to achieve cardiovascular fitness but not so fast that it's too strenuous. A person's target zone varies with his age. The way to figure out yours is to determine your maximal attainable heart rate, which is the point where the heart is unable to beat any faster—that is, where it is unable to transport any more oxygen to the muscles to create the energy to continue the exercising."

"And the idea is I'm to exercise to the point where I get up to that maximal whosis?"

"No, the idea is to get to a heart rate between seventy and eighty-five percent of that maximal attainable rate. That's a person's target zone. Below seventy percent you achieve only limited fitness, although right now any exercise you do is of benefit, since you've been pretty much bedridden. And eighty-five percent is the top."

"That's like red-lining on the r.p.m.'s, huh? Is it dangerous if I go past that?"

"That's a factor, but also exercise beyond that point won't bring you any additional benefit. There's a point where, in spite of our best efforts, the heart and circulation can't deliver more oxygen to the tissues. And we can't exercise long on that level or above it without approaching exhaustion. That's the maximal attainable heart rate."

"What's my target zone?"

"Well, let's figure it out. For someone at your age, forty-four, in good health, the maximum heartbeat after the most strenuous exercise you could do safely has been calculated to be 176 beats per minute. O.K., the target zone is between seventy and eighty-five percent of that. That's between . . ."

Frank computed quickly on the sketch pad. ". . . 123 and 150 beats per minute. That's my target zone."

"And that's what we'll be aiming to get to with the exercises."

"What kind of exercises do I get to do? Besides tennis, of course." He sneaked a look at me.

I pulled a booklet out of my bag. *"Exercise Your Way to*

Fitness and Heart Health. The latest findings for the cardiac. It's written very clearly and simply." I handed it to him.

"By Dr. Lenore Zohman," he read. "By a dame, huh?"

"One of the leading specialists in exercise therapy for heart patients and people who don't want to be heart patients."

"Not bad looking," he commented judiciously. A folded typewritten sheet fell out from between the pages. "What's this?"

"That's a list I had typed out of various exercises you can start with during the first months of your recovery program."

Frank scanned the sheet like a man reading his son's bad report card.

"Calisthenics!" he groaned.

"Right. Incidentally, I'll periodically be giving you a cardiac stress test in my office. Then we'll know the maximum stress your heart can safely take when you exercise."

He was barely listening. "I've always hated calisthenics."

"Well, this is one program where substitutes are permitted. How about jumping rope? It exercises both arms and legs. It increases coordination, endurance, and stamina."

"Not my dish of tea. How about weight lifting? It's something I always thought I might like to try."

"Not your dish of tea. In the first place, it's isometric."

"Meaning?"

"Weight lifting squeezes the blood vessels, letting less blood pass instead of more. Any exercise that tenses the muscles—like weight lifting or push-ups or pole vaulting or discus throwing—will develop your muscles, but it'll do little for your cardiovascular fitness. Isometric exercises won't help rehabilitate your heart."

Frank was getting restive. "Well, Christ, are there any exercises that are any *fun* that I can do?"

"Isotonic or dynamic exercise is what you want. That's exercise that's rhythmic, repetitive, and involves motion. That kind of exercise helps make the blood flow through your body."

He nodded. "O.K., isotonic . . ."

"And aerobic."

"Now what?"

"That merely means any rhythmic exercise that can be sustained for a fairly decent period of time without exhausting you or making you breathless. Sprinting, for instance, is not aerobic, nor are acrobatics. Ideal isotonic and aerobic exercises are things like walking, swimming . . ."

Frank nodded dolefully as he picked up the list. ". . . jogging, calisthenics, jumping rope . . . everything I find really monotonous."

"Because there's no competition in it?"

"What's wrong with enjoying competing? Come on, Doc, let's face it. Without competition, exercise is a bore."

"I agree with you one hundred percent. A competitor makes it a game, and a game keeps the physical activity going. Well, now, just think what your real competition is: a second heart attack."

Frank gave a start.

"And the game you're in is *survival.* So, the more closely you adhere to the rules, the more religiously you do your exercises, the more points you're going to pile up to survive."

Frank was quiet as he read the typewritten exercise schedule again. "I like swimming."

"That's a terrific exercise. It uses every part of your body without the pounding you get from jogging, for instance.

Some doctors don't believe in jogging for cardiac patients, but there's no one I know of against swimming. Another good one is bicycling."

"Bicycling? Forget it," said Frank. "I never learned how."

"Does your son ride a bike?"

"It seems to me there were years I used to buy him one every Christmas. He kept outgrowing them or smashing them or getting them stolen."

"But he does ride."

"Yeah, I suppose so."

"Good. Then he can teach you."

Frank bridled a little. "My son teach me?"

"It's also a way of growing, Frank. Listening to your children. And I imagine it would give your son a lot of pleasure. Being able to teach his father a skill."

Frank gave me a rueful look. "You really are out to redesign my future, aren't you? Frank & Family will reopen shortly under a new policy."

"Business not going on as usual during alterations," I suggested.

"Look for our sensational new family style."

"Frank, you may come out of all this with a happier way of life."

"I thought I was pretty happy the old way."

"The new way may last a lot longer."

"Knock wood. Harold, level with me. Do I *ever* get to play tennis again?"

"Let me put it this way, Frank. Tennis is your luxury. Luxuries come last and you've got to be able to afford them. You do your exercises and stick to the diet I'll give you and you'll be able to afford it."

"O.K. When?"

I gave in. "You'll probably start batting a ball over the net to your wife. Does she play tennis?"

"She's lousy."

"Good. It means you'll be able to start tennis slowly and gradually build up, instead of playing in spurts. Besides it'll help her game. You'll start in about three months . . ."

"If everything goes smoothly." Frank imitated my demeanor.

I smiled. "If everything goes smoothly you should be back to your regular game in about five to six months."

"Good enough," said Frank grudgingly, folding the exercise schedule I had given him carefully. "Now tell me about my diet."

"Not today." I patted his shoulder. "I've got to get back to the office."

"O.K." His face took on a look of solicitude. "Say, Harold . . ."

"Yes?"

"You know you're looking a bit peaked. Why don't you lie down for about an hour after lunch, then take a half hour jog, then . . ."

"I'll begin the jogging right now," I said—and trotted eight steps to the door.

9. Resurrection

"I phoned Joan this morning at her office like I always do," said Allen Seberling, who was himself on the phone to me. "She sounded out of breath. So I say to her, kidding, 'Hey, Joan, what's with you? Sounds like you're having sex or something.' She says, 'What the hell are you talking about, Allen?' I say, 'The way you're panting so hard.' Well, she gets real ticked off and gives me hell. Finally she admits she's been short of breath all morning and all day yesterday."

I hadn't heard from Joan Seberling (or Ms. Joan Ellen) since her last visit almost eleven months earlier, when I'd first detected her borderline hypertension. I had scheduled subsequent monthly visits to check her blood pressure, but she did not show for her first appointment nor did she phone to cancel it. When Nanci, my secretary, called her office to check, Joan's secretary said she knew nothing of the appointment, and after a minute came back on the phone to convey her boss's apologies: "Ms. Ellen forgot to tell me to put it on her calendar, and then it slipped her mind entirely."

A new appointment was scheduled a week later. Joan didn't keep that one either. Her secretary phoned that an office emergency had come up and there was no way Ms. Ellen could get away; she would phone tomorrow to make a new appointment. She didn't phone. At the end of the week I took a hand and phoned myself. Joan was in Chicago. She would phone me on her return, which would be within the week. There was no return phone call and I didn't call her again, although I did drop her a note asking her to schedule an appointment. I learned long ago that trying to corral a reluctant patient is an idle pursuit.

My surmise was that she felt justified in postponing her follow-up visit because she considered her symptoms to be minor, and if she stayed away long enough, she could convince herself that my warning of possible trouble was absurd. It would take more alarming manifestations than rapid heart beats and cold hands and feet when under tension to bring her back to my office.

Now, many months later, her ex-husband was on the phone telling me of her current physical disturbance.

"What does it mean, Doc, when someone has been short of breath two days running?"

"It could be one or a combination of things."

"For instance?"

"Allen, I can't diagnose on the basis of a single symptom related to me on the phone by a second party. Why don't you tell Joan to call me?"

"I did and she told me not to tell her what to do. Said

she's had sixteen years of me telling her and that was enough. So I said I'll be glad to call you myself and she told me to mind my own damned business and hung up on me. You know she hates to take orders. She had a very domineering father she hated, you know, and I told her once it was her mother's fault for not standing up to him. Boy, did she blow a gasket!"

"Many patients don't really want to find out what's wrong. Some people consider themselves immortal almost, and refuse to believe that they can get sick or die. Alan, call her, tell her you spoke with me, and have her give me a call at the office immediately, will you?"

"I've *tried* calling her, but her secretary keeps saying she's in meetings, which means she doesn't want to talk to me." His voice became supplicatory. "Say, Doc, could you . . . is it possible you would phone her about this?"

"Of course I'll call her."

Ms. Ellen wasn't in. Would Dr. Karpman care to leave his phone number? Yes, Dr. Karpman would. In fact, the doctor would also like to leave his schedule for the rest of the day, with phone numbers at each stop-off, and he would like his call returned as soon as possible.

I heard from Ms. Ellen about two hours later. I was in a hospital visiting Jenny Rosen. This was a year after her attack of heart failure. She had continued with her daily dosage of digitalis, but she had ignored my instructions and was now back in the hospital with a case of digitalis poisoning.

"I was taking a pill every morning like you told me," she explained. "It made me feel so much better that sometimes when I was tired I'd take another one."

"And maybe a third one and sometimes a fourth one."

"Sometimes, so what's such a calamity?"

"I'll tell you. You were vomiting these past two weeks. You had palpitations. You almost blacked out. You lost weight. And now you're in the hospital . . ."

"Well, at least I did lose weight. That's what you wanted me to do." Like many patients, Jenny had long since discovered humor as a defense against the scolding of the parent of old age—the physician.

"Of course, taking too much digitalis will make you lose weight. The same way as you can lose a headache by shooting yourself in the leg," I said severely, "do you remember what I explained to you about digitalis the night you had your congestive failure?"

"You said, first, the heart wasn't pumping good so the blood was jamming up . . . like a stopped-up toilet—"

"That's not what I'm talking about . . ."

"Oh, no. Like in a bathtub, excuse me . . ."

"The important thing I told you, Jenny, was that to keep your heart pumping steadily you were to take a certain amount of digitalis every day, no more, no less."

"I remember now."

"Too much digitalis can make you sick or even kill you. Digitalis isn't like aspirin, Jenny."

"Yes, Dr. Karpman," she said, subdued.

"If you take too much digitalis, it can build up in the bloodstream and actually poison the system. That's why you lost your appetite and why you were vomiting. You could easily have had bad heart complications, Jenny—"

"God forbid! He should punish me if I ever take one thing you don't order me to take, Dr. Karpman . . ."

The bedside phone rang. "That's probably David," she beamed, picking it up. "He called twice already. Hello?"

She looked surprised. "Yes, he's right here." She held out the receiver to me. "It's from a Miss Ellen."

"Oh, yes. Do you mind if I talk to her on your phone?"

"Be my guest." She settled back against her pillow to listen.

I took the phone as far from the bed as I could and turned my back. "How are you, Joan?"

"This is Joan Ellen's secretary," came an unsteady voice. "She had a heart attack here in the office. It was so sudden. She asked me to call you. I had your numbers and—"

"Where is she now?"

"Mayflower Hospital. A fire department ambulance took her there."

"Thank you. I'll get back to you."

I hung up, phoned my secretary, and asked her to read me my appointments for the rest of the day. I told her which patients to reschedule and which to refer to my associates in the office who covered for me in emergencies. As for anyone already in the waiting room, I instructed her to explain that I had a hospital emergency and they could either wait or see one of the other doctors.

No patients enjoy such rearrangements, but I have found most surprisingly understanding. As one elderly gentleman once put it to me, "Whenever your secretary tells me you'll be delayed because of a hospital emergency I think, 'Thank God I'm not the emergency,' and I relax and wait." "And that kind of thinking," I had told him, "is possibly what helps to keep you from becoming an emergency."

I hung up and apologized to Jenny for monopolizing her phone. "Oh, no," she said, exhilarated, "it was like listening to Marcus Welby. What's the matter with the poor girl?"

"She didn't follow her doctor's instructions," I said pointedly, as I left.

When I arrived at the Mayflower Hospital I found Joan on an examination table in the Coronary Care emergency room. A cardiac monitor with a pulse rate meter was already transmitting from the electrodes taped on her chest and legs.

The charge nurse said Joan had been delivered by the rescue squad in extreme distress, with a squeezing pain in her upper chest, her breathing shallow and rapid. The doctor on duty in the hospital's emergency room had sent her right up to the Coronary Care Unit.

"We've given her ten milligrams of morphine for the pain," the nurse said.

"What's her blood pressure?"

"O.K. 134 over 82. She's very upset about being here."

Slightly sedated by the morphine, Joan insisted she was not having a heart attack. "You know . . . one third of the people taken to hospitals like this . . . to Coronary Care Units, turn out to be victims of . . . of—"

"Indigestion or other things," I finished. I opened my bag and started taking out my stethescope. "Yes, I read the same article in last Sunday's paper. Now, don't talk anymore. Just rest."

"But if it's just indigestion," she said, indignantly, "why should I get rushed into a hospital and then . . ."

At that moment, as though in answer, she rolled up her eyes and lost consciousness.

The cardiac monitor sounded a piercing beep. A light on it flashed red indicating Joan's heart had stopped beating.

Her lips and fingernails began taking on a bluish tinge. Her face was ashen white.

"Nurse! Hit the Code Blue button!" I snapped.

The nurse punched a button on the wall, activating the two-foot wide timer over the bed which went up to ten minutes. Then she quickly dialed the special number on the phone.

Almost immediately the loudspeakers all over the hospital began squawking. *"Code Blue, CCU. Code Blue, CCU."*

I tried to locate a pulse in Joan's neck and then groin while simultaneously listening to her heart through the stethescope. There was no pulse or heart action.

Ostensibly she was dead, although her pupils had not yet dilated, indicating brain damage hadn't yet occurred. If circulation was not restored in four or five minutes there would be damage to the brain that would be irreversible.

"I'm starting closed chest resuscitation!" I said to the nurse. "Lower the bed!"

As the bed came down, I slipped a board that was kept in the CCU under Joan's back in order to make her body more rigid. I needed all the leverage I could get during the closed chest resuscitation.

I placed the heal of my right hand on her lower chest—in the midline portion of the sternum—and covered it with my left hand. Elbows locked, I thrust down hard, putting my weight behind each thrust, then letting up. The procedure isn't easy; there must be sixty thrusts a minute.

Even with the board and lowered bed I couldn't get sufficient purchase. So I climbed onto the bed, straddled Joan's limp form, and continued pushing against the breastbone, yelling like the coxswain of a rowing crew.

"One . . . two . . . three . . . four . . . five—*breathe* . . . !"

That was for the nurse. She had put a pillow under Joan's neck, tilted her head back and pried her mouth open to pull the tongue back and open the airway to the lungs. Now she was administering air with a positive pressure bag, pumping air in just as Joan's chest expanded at the end of every fifth chest compression.

Closed chest resuscitation squeezes the heart like a balloon. Because the breast bone above the heart is hinged, each down-thrust pushes the heart against the spine, compressing it, and each release lets it resume its normal shape. The heart is thus being pumped like a bellows. At the end of each fifth thrust, as the hand comes up off the chest and the heart and lungs are permitted to expand, mouth-to-mouth respiration or other mechanical methods of artificial respiration are used to force air or oxygen into the lungs. Thus, there is sort of a forced feeding of the cardiovascular system and, most importantly, of the brain, which must have oxygen available to it continuously to prevent death.

Seconds after the nurse had sounded the Code Blue button, the members of the hospital's specially trained resuscitation squad—medical house staff members, inhalation therapists, an EKG technician, an anesthesiologist, two CCU nurses—began pouring into the room. Within fifty seconds of Joan's losing consciousness, according to the clock, the entire team was there.

Relieving the nurse, the inhalation therapist placed a small rubber airway in Joan's open mouth, and administered 100 percent oxygen down her throat after each fifth thrust. The anesthesiologist removed the rubber airway and inserted an endotrachial tube which opened a pathway to send oxygen directly into the airway to the lungs.

"Start an infusion of five percent dextrose and water in the right arm," I told the I.V. nurse as I continued performing the resuscitation. I then asked the medication nurse to prepare medications I might need in the next few minutes.

During all this activity—performed as smoothly and intricately as a ballet performance—the EKG technician unobtrusively hooked up a cardiograph machine, thus clearly demonstrating what I suspected was the cause of Joan's collapse, a form of arrhythmia known as ventricular fibrillation.

Arrhythmia is pretty much what the word sounds like— "out of rhythm." Normally the chambers of the heart pump in consecutive one-two order. To push blood through the entire cardiovascular system, the pumping system is triggered in sequence by a series of natural electrical pacemakers in the heart. Sometimes, a coronary attack will make these pacemakers go out of sync, like spark plugs firing out of order in an automobile engine.

Joan's form of arrhythmia was ventricular fibrillation, a particularly deadly kind. The left ventricle of the heart, responsible for pumping blood through the entire body, suddenly stops beating rhythmically and its action is reduced to a helpless, rapid quiver. It is like an electrical machine in short circuit, crackling and sparking, ineffective. On the electrocardiograph, the stylus registers this condition as wildly wiggling lines.

The timer over the bed indicated more than two minutes had passed. In that time we had managed (1) to keep her circulation going, (2) to send oxygenated blood to all parts of the body, (3) to discover what caused the circulation to collapse. Our attempt now would be to restore it and prevent Joan's brain from suffering fatal damage from oxygen starvation. For the moment we were in control.

"Defibrillators," I called out. "And give her one amp of bicarb. I.V. stat." Circulatory arrest produces certain biochemical changes in the body which are temporarily corrected by intermittently injecting an alkalyzing solution, sodium bicarbonate until the normal circulation is reestablished.

"One amp of bicarb," repeated the medication nurse. She swiftly found the medication and infused it into the I.V.

tubing connecting the bottle of dextrose and water to a vein in Joan's arm.

The defibrillators, looking like a pair of long-handled small frying pans, were handed to me by the charge nurse. Applying them to Joan's chest, I sent a high-voltage electric shock through her heart. Defibrillation is like giving a person in hysterics a sharp slap. When the heart, quivering ineffectively in ventricular fibrillation, is given an electrical shock, it stops dead for a moment, then hopefully resumes pumping effectively.

The shock made Joan jerk upwards like a fish on a line, then fall back on the bed.

The charge nurse felt for her pulse. She shook her head. The EKG monitor continued to show a disorganized heart action.

"No show," the EKG technician said.

The pulse volume with each thrust on the chest decreased, the blood pressure was dropping.

We had a little more than a minute to go.

I could feel my own pulse pounding in my temples. "O.K., let's try again."

I applied a second shock. The body again sprang upward. Then, after the longest moment of silence, the EKG scope showed a normal rhythm. A minute later Joan opened her eyes.

"Second shot was a winner," the resident doctor said happily.

The cardiac monitor had resumed beeping and the EKG showed a steady weave as Joan's heart settled down to a normal beat. I told the medication nurse to give Joan a solution containing lidocaine, to stave off further arrhythmia.

When I finally left the CCU, greatly exhilarated and

somewhat exhausted, I passed Allen Seberling as I headed for the elevator. He pounced on me.

"Doctor, what's happened?"

"How did you learn about it so fast?"

"Her secretary phoned me. For God's sake, how is she?"

"She had a coronary. Hopefully, the damage will be minimal, but it was complicated by an arrhythmia, ventricular fibrillation. But she responded to therapy and pulled through beautifully."

"What do you mean—'pulled through?' A cousin of mine once had a fibrillation and it wasn't even serious. How come this one is?"

We both got in the elevator. "Allen, let's have a fast cup of coffee in the restaurant. I'll answer all your questions there before I head back to the office, O.K.?"

Allen's eyes were riveted to me as I took my first sip of coffee.

"This cousin of yours had fibrillation that wasn't serious, you say . . ."

"It wasn't, Doc. She had to take some drugs—digitalis and stuff . . ."

"Did she have atrial fibrillation?"

"That's right. Atrial."

"Well, Joan had ventricular fibrillation. That's much, much more serious." On a napkin I sketched the heart with its four spaces. "The heart, as you know, is composed of four chambers."

Allen looked at it. "Biology One was a long time back, but I still remember that. The two top chambers are the auricles, the bottom ones are the ventricles, right?"

"They don't call them auricles anymore. They're called atria, Latin for cavity or waiting room. The left and right atria are chambers where the blood goes before being pumped into the ventricles and from there, depending on whether it's the right ventricle or the left one, either is carried into the lungs or into the entire body. The ventricles have thick muscled walls and are the real pumps of the heart. The right ventricle pumps blood through the lungs."

"And the left one pumps blood through the body. It's coming back to me. The left ventricle is the real powerhouse."

"Exactly. Now the chambers all pump in order," I illustrated with arrows through the heart chambers I had drawn, "so the blood moves in a steady stream. They're synchronized, so to speak. Now what happened to your cousin was that her atria became unsynchronized, started to beat rapidly and wildly, and lost sync."

"How could that happen?"

"Well, the heart has a number of natural pacemakers buried in its muscle walls that control the pumping of each of the chambers. Like a line-up of spark plugs firing in split-second consecutive order. Sometimes what happens with certain people like your cousin is that for a variety of reasons, one or two of those spark plugs misfire or fire out of turn."

"They lose sync."

"Exactly. Now when a natural pacemaker goes out of wack—say, one of the atria—the atrial pumping can go from seventy-five beats a minute to four or even five hundred a minute. It's not pumping anymore; it's just twitching or quivering, with an occasional beat coming through."

"And then the heart stops?"

"Oh, no. Not with an atrial fibrillation."

"But it can't pump blood into the left ventricle."

"Its pumping has never been of major importance to the

circulation. The atriums are more important as collecting chambers for blood. It's the ventricles that keep the blood going. So the blood is pushed through the ineffective atrial chambers from behind, so to speak, into the ventricles, which are still pumping along at a good rate. Even if the ventricular rate was very fast, it could usually be slowed with digitalis. So your cousin felt weak, felt how irregular the heartbeat was. But at least there was enough blood going through the system to keep her going. Atrial fibrillation is not a matter of life or death."

"But ventricular fibrillation is?"

"Figure it out. As you said, the left ventricle is the powerhouse. It pumps blood through the entire circulatory system except for the lungs. When it goes into fibrillation and starts quivering instead of pumping, *no* blood at all is being pumped out into the body. And if the brain is deprived of oxygen for more than four or five minutes, it is irreparably damaged; in five or six minutes, it may be dead. That's why it is so important to get help fast when there's a suspicion of a coronary. A person should get to the hospital immediately because that is where these serious complications can be rapidly detected and, more important, effectively treated. Fortunately, Joan was already in the Coronary Care Unit when it happened. That fibrillation came up fast but we detected it within seconds and we had the instruments on hand to give her heart an electric shock and get the rhythm back to normal. If she had been in her office or in the car she would have been in serious trouble. That's why it's important to get to the hospital *fast* when a heart attack is suspected."

"What's to keep it from happening again?"

"Well, we've found that if we put minute amounts of

lidocaine, the stuff your dentist uses to numb your tooth before drilling, or other drugs that reduce the irritability of the injured heart muscles, into the bloodstream it will usually cause the abnormal heart rhythms to diminish, thereby decreasing the threat of ventricular fibrillation."

The waitress arrived with the check. Allen covered it and simultaneously reached for the napkin on which I had drawn the heart. "I'm buying your medical drawing," he said.

For the first five days after her heart had resumed beating regularly, Joan lay in bed in the Coronary Care Unit in a state of apathy. She would acknowledge my daily arrival with only a distant nod, rarely look at me as she curtly answered my questions, never asked any questions herself, and submitted to all tests, injections, and intravenous feedings with complete indifference.

Coming out of the CCU one day, I found Allen in the corridor, who had already seen Joan during the time permitted relatives of patients. I had talked the hospital into stretching a point and treating Allen as Joan's nearest relative. After all, he was more responsible than anyone for the fact that his ex wife was alive.

"She won't even look at me when I'm standing right next to her bed," he said mournfully as we walked to the elevator. "Any time I ask if she wants me to do anything, she just shakes her head. The only time she nods yes is when I ask if she wants me to go away. Maybe she hates me."

"Maybe she hates me, too."

Allen gave me a startled look.

"Actually," I went on, "she doesn't hate either of us. I'd say she's having a deep mental readjustment. A coronary is brutal enough, but when you have it accompanied by ventricular fibrillation, it takes time to come out of that trauma. Sometimes a lot of time."

"She hates me," Allen said stubbornly. We stood waiting for the elevator.

"Allen, how did you find out that Joan had a heart attack?"

"I told you. Her secretary phoned me at the office. I was down at the hospital like a shot."

"The secretary phoned you on Joan's instructions, right?"

"I guess so."

"Do you think a woman having a heart attack, headed for the hospital, would tell her secretary to give that information to a man she hates?"

Allen was silent.

"You know, I've always thought it interesting that the last name she uses at work is Ellen and your first name is Allen."

"Yeah. Funny, I've never asked her about that." He seemed to be thinking hard.

The down elevator arrived and I checked my watch. "I've got time for a fast coffee. This one's on me."

"Thanks, Doc, but..." he hit the UP button, looking embarrassed. "Guess I'd better go upstairs. Maybe she'll feel better and want to see me. If I'm up there, you know, maybe they'll call me."

He gave me a wave as the doors closed.

By the sixth day, Joan's physical condition had improved to the point where she could be moved to a regular hospital room. When I came in for the first time, she was sitting up in bed, reading a book. She closed it as I came in, but gave no smile in answer to my greeting.

"You're feeling better," I told her.

"Is that what it says on your charts?"

"Oh, no. There's color in your face today."

"Oh, is there?" Her face lit up with small triumph. "That's make-up. I put on lipstick and a little rouge."

"I know," I smiled, "and when a woman patient starts using make-up it means she's feeling better."

She looked discomfited, then fixed me with a reproachful look. "You know, you could have warned me."

"About what?"

"About what happened. All you told me was that I had a little high blood pressure. You didn't tell me I could have a heart attack."

"I didn't know it was going to happen."

"What did you know?"

I drew up a chair next to the bed and sat down. A seated doctor is much more relaxing to talk to than a standing one.

"Joan, you came to me eleven months ago with symptoms of functional vasospasms and borderline hypertension. I explained to you that these conditions are hardly dangerous in themselves, but could be a warning that you were under a lot of pressure and tension. Once you learn that, you should make a solid effort to control that pressure and tension. You should examine yourself, find out what creates the major tensions in your life, change the patterns of their thinking, learn to relax, to think differently. If your doctor recommends it, you should go on a diet to reduce cholesterol and lose weight, and you should stop smoking. Often the hypertension will disappear, if the tension and pressure of living is lessened."

"You didn't tell me all this could happen in less than a year."

"Joan, would you say that an adult has the responsibility

for all decisions in relation to their health, and that the physician is mainly their advisor?"

"Yes," she said thoughtfully, "I would say that."

"Well, eleven months ago when you consulted me, I told you you had incipient high blood pressure. I told you that people who have high blood pressure run a greater risk of developing heart attacks, strokes, and kidney problems. I told you some changes in your lifestyle might eliminate the hypertension and that you should report to me monthly. You didn't. Now let me ask you—why didn't you?"

Joan had the grace to blush. "After I'd seen you, I met someone who had the same kind of problem I had, and they had had them twenty years and they never went to see a doctor and their blood pressure was fine. I *know* they weren't lying to me."

"I'm sure they weren't. Sometimes it stays dormant for years, or never advances."

"Why?"

"We don't know. The natural history or progression of many illnesses varies considerably, depending on the person. But frequently, if you depressurize your life, watch your diet, and so on, you can prevent or eliminate high blood pressure.

"How did my heart get affected?"

"Hypertension tends to make atherosclerosis come on earlier in life. One of your coronary arteries, a small one, finally clotted up and closed."

"Is that why my heart stopped?"

"No. One can have a massive coronary and the heart will beat steadily through it, or, on the other hand, one can have a tiny coronary artery occlusion like you did and the heartbeat goes out of wack like it did for you."

"Why does it come with some cases and not in others?"

"We don't know for sure . . ."

"If you ask me, you doctors have more ignorance than anything," she snapped.

I sighed. "Well, we're trying to reduce that ignorance. For instance, before World War II a patient with significant hypertension could look forward to a few sick years probably ending in a stroke or possibly in kidney or heart failure. Now we have the drugs to control hypertension to bring the blood pressure down and allow patients to lead a normal life with a normal life expectancy. Or take your heart arrest in the emergency room. If you had had that ventricular fibrillation on an examining table twenty years ago, all the doctors and nurses of that day couldn't have saved you."

Joan blushed. "I'm sorry," she said slowly, "I had no business saying doctors are ignorant."

"But they are, in certain areas. Maybe less ignorant than twenty years ago but, hopefully, a lot more than twenty years from now."

She was shaking her head. "No, I'm sorry to be so bitchy, it's just that . . ." Her eyes glistened with tears. "I'm so discouraged."

"Why? You've been doing very well, and you'll be out of here in less than two weeks and back at your job in less than a month."

"What job?"

That gave me pause. I'd forgotten about the president in Chicago who disliked women in executive jobs. "You mean you were fired?"

"Not yet, but under the circumstances I really can't blame J.G. if he does fire me."

"Under what circumstances?"

"Oh, come on, Doctor, let's be realistic. I'm damaged goods now."

"Like hell you are! O.K., you had a small coronary occlusion. But it was very small, and there's a scar on your heart now that's shortly going to be stronger than the tissue it replaced. You can do your work every bit as good as before and if you follow the regime I will lay out for you in terms of diet, exercise, and recreation, you'll probably be able to do your job even better."

"Thank you, Doctor." She smiled ruefully. "If only there was some way to convey that to J.G."

"I can tell you how one of my other patients conveyed it to his boss."

"How?"

"He bearded the lion in his den. He flew to the company headquarters in Omaha and had a talk with the chairman of the board. He said, 'You think I'm an invalid because I've had a coronary. The facts of the case are I'm not. I'm equipped to be as good or better executive than I was before. I know just what you're worried about.' And he listed the worries, one, two, three. 'One, I can't cope with my responsibilities. Two, I might drop dead on the job. Three, I'll need special treatment. All dead wrong,' he told his boss."

Joan was listening raptly.

"He told him exactly what I've told you. His heart was stronger and as a result of losing weight, going on a health diet, exercising regularly, stopping smoking, learning to handle tension instead of tension handling him, and because of the incentive to *show* he was better than before, he would be a more alert, reliable, and conscientious employee than he had ever been before. He kept his job and he's been promoted since."

"Horray for our side." She smiled, then added thoughtfully, "You know when I go to beard J.G. in Chicago, I th.nk I'll propose a new course in my school: three hours a week of instruction in physical fitness, with emphasis on preventing cardiac trouble—you know, a regime of diet, exercise, relaxation, counter-tension. It's not a bad idea and it'.l show that old bastard I'm still on the ball, right?"

"Well, it certainly ought to help spike the guns of that ambitious assistant of yours—you know, the one who's gunning for your job."

There was no question about her blushing now. "You mean Brady?" She cleared her throat. "I forgot to tell you he came to visit me yesterday and suggested I take out a policy with an insurance company that writes policies for people who've recovered from coronaries. He says a lot of companies do that."

"Brady told you about it?"

"He said a policy like that would impress J.G. The idea being if an insurance company is willing to bet on me, why shouldn't J.G.?"

"Excellent idea! But I thought Brady was trying to get your job."

She looked embarrassed. "I guess I was wrong about him. Maybe it was all that tension building up in me. Now, Doctor, you're sure I'll be able to go back to that job?"

"Most coronary patients get back to their former jobs. So if that's what you enjoy doing, by all means go back to it when you're recovered. But I suggest you no longer treat it like it was your whole life. Your livelihood, yes. But don't confuse it with your life."

"What else *is* my life?"

"That's your next project, Joan. Find interests that can absorb you."

"You mean like men?"

"If interest in men can reduce your absorption in your

job, then that's the best medicine you can take for your heart."

"I don't know if that would work for me," Joan shrugged. "Oh, I've had my share of affairs, but I've found that every time I go to bed with a man he starts trying to run my life."

"Are you sure you don't start the relationship with the assumption that that's going to happen?"

She looked at me sharply. "You mean that I'm prejudiced in advance? That's a male chauvinist comment, and quite ridiculous. If there's one thing I pride myself on, Doctor, it's being clear-eyed and objective, especially about men."

"Except for Brady, of course."

She didn't answer. I looked at my watch and stood up. "You're coming along fine. I'll see you tomorrow."

The next morning Joan was reading a book when I came in, but this time she smiled to me in greeting. "I'm glad you came when you did," she said. "I just read something I want you to hear." She held up the book so I could read the title, *Hey, God, What Should I Do Now?* by Jess Lair, Ph.D. and Jacqueline Carey Lair.

"This guy was an advertising man who got a massive coronary and then turned his life around—went back to school and eventually became a psychology professor. Listen to what he says about heart attacks."

She opened the book and read. " 'I see heart attacks as coming from a heart that is slowly shriveling up from lack of love. The physical activities that precipitate the attack are more a symptom of the problem than the problem itself. But most doctors can do so little about feelings and are so afraid of feelings themselves that they concentrate on the patient's physical symptoms and activity.' " She lowered the book and looked at me mischievously. "What do you think of that, Doctor?"

I sat down. "Well, I'm afraid I've got to throw myself at the mercy of the court. I don't know. Love is a healing factor, but its effectiveness simply can't be accurately measured. Tender Loving Care is accepted medical therapy, and many cardiologists believe that the love of a spouse or partner is an important psychological element in a heart victim's recovery. I don't think doctors are necessarily afraid of feeling. In fact, they're frequently deeply affected by their patient's illnesses. However, we are scientists and are more comfortable with proven facts. Lack of love and the associated anxiety and depression cannot be excluded as a contributing factor in some heart attacks. Still, I'm certainly not ready to proclaim love as a coronary preventative."

Joan's eyes twinkled. "How about setting up a Masters and Johnson type laboratory and testing out the theory there?"

"I don't think sex was in the mind of your author-psychologist when he was talking about love."

"You weren't excluding it when you suggested I try a man as a cure for hypertension, were you?" Joan giggled. She was enjoying pulling my leg.

"Now that was a specific prescription for a specific patient. A great cardiologist once said 'It is more important to know what sort of person had the disease than to know what sort of disease the person had.'"

Joan stopped smiling.

"My God," she said, "that's exactly what I've been wondering about since yesterday, Doctor. What sort of a person I really am. So I've been putting myself through the wringer all night."

She swallowed exactly as she had done the previous day before making the confession about Brady. "Maybe I *am* prejudiced against men. My father was always bossing my poor mother around, yelling at her a lot. Maybe I figure all men are like that basically, so I jump down their throat as soon as they open their mouths."

"You must have been through an agonizing reappraisal last night."

"It wasn't that agonizing. I've suspected myself a long time. It was just a question of admitting my hypocrisy, and that Brady business made it impossible not to. But last night I dug deeper. I thought about my poor mother and I had to admit she enjoyed provoking my father into yelling, she enjoyed being bossed around, looking like a martyr at the same time. I finally realized that my poor father was jumping through her hoops. That was an eye-opener!"

"Well, better late than never."

"No, it's inexcusable. Lots of times in our marriage Allen would try to point that out to me and, boy, would I jump down *his* throat! You know why I didn't want to see it? Because there's a lot of my mother in me. Like dropping hints about not feeling well to Allen so he would nag me into seeing you. I really did want to see a doctor, but I always wanted to feel I was being bullied into it." She shook her head. "When I think of all I've put that poor guy through!"

"You're getting quite a perspective."

"Just beginning, Doctor."

Later, as I waited in front of the elevators, Allen stepped out of one. His face brightened.

"Hi, Doc." He looked at me anxiously. "How is she?"

"She's improving, Allen. So go in and enjoy."

10. Eat, Drink, and Be Healthy

Frank waved a hand as I entered his hospital room. Dressed in blue pajamas edged in scarlet, he was sprawled on top of his bed, a newspaper in front of him, talking on the phone. ". . . O.K., Bert, the doctor just came in and I gotta hang up. Just quick read me back my prices. . . . Hold it, on that one make it a ten; I'm positive we got a winner there. O.K., that's it. Talk to you at five."

He hung up and gave me that slightly mocking smile I was beginning to regard as standard equipment.

"Are you running your business on the phone?"

"Nope. That was my bookie."

"I didn't know you played the ponies."

"I didn't until you told me I was too competitive for my own good and I should find some recreation. So I figured I'd bet on the horses and let them do the competing."

"Very funny."

"Nothing wrong with it, is there, Doc?"

"Those are pretty classy pajamas, Frank."

"You didn't answer my question, Doc. Is there anything wrong with me playing the ponies to relax me?"

"*If* it relaxes you. But as I see it, all you're doing is substituting horses for dresses. You're still competing. Is it relaxing you? You're the only one who can answer that."

Frank thought a moment. "You know, Harold, this morning I was handicapping," he gestured at the newspaper which I could see was a racing form, "and suddenly I felt the same excitement comes up in me when we're getting the new spring line ready for the buyers. Naah, it's a busman's holiday." He crumpled the paper and threw it in the wastebasket. "Bye, bye, bookie. I'll take up bird watching."

"I can't believe it," I said. "Frank Justin giving in without an argument."

He grinned. "Today I'm a pussycat. After all, in two days I'll be flying outa this coop."

"You're looking forward to leaving?"

"Well, of course! What do you think?"

"You'd be surprised how many patients are afraid to leave the security of a hospital. It's as though they're back in the womb and they're in no hurry to get out of it this time."

"That's hard to believe."

"Believe it."

"I do. It's like when I was drafted and sent to Germany. When my year was up, I couldn't wait to get out, but there was a couple of guys who'd found a home in the army. They're probably still in."

"That's not quite the same thing. Everybody looks for a home somewhere. But when you want to stay in a hospital because you feel safer in one even after your heart is well enough for you to be out, then you're on the way to becoming a cardiac cripple."

"That I'm not."

"You want to get back into action, huh? Feel good enough to play a game of tennis?"

"A game? Hell, a couple of sets."

"O.K., let's talk about that. Recovering from an illness is really a joy. Every day you're getting stronger, capable of doing more than you did yesterday. It's like a kid growing up. Nothing sweeter than the first day you can walk under your own power or ride a two wheeler or hit a homer. Only now you're not a kid growing up, you're a convalescent who's been improving in an institution where they treat you like you're made of glass. Now you're starting to get the feeling that you could get right out and knock off a set of tennis. But the truth is, it'll take you a lot of exercise and toning up before you can even serve a ball over the net. You've been at virtually complete bed rest for almost three weeks. You're out of shape."

Frank gave me a wry look. "What are you trying to do, Harold—spoil my day?"

"Frank, you're going to be bushed for at least a couple of days after you get home."

Frank shrugged. "I wasn't expecting to dance the polka right off."

"I doubt if you'll even do a two-step. Chances are you'll want to head right for bed. After three weeks in a hospital, a simple thing like returning home can be awfully fatiguing."

"Suppose I fool you and feel great when I get home?"

"I still recommend you take it easy for a day or two. The first few days should be a continuation of your last few days here at the hospital. Rest at least an hour after each meal. Do all your walking inside the house. If it's warm, you can sit outside in the shade. When I start you on your daily walks out of the house—"

". . . Take a buddy."

"That's not what I was going to say."

Frank wagged his head. "There I go finishing sentences."

"At least you're getting to be aware of it. Now, when you take your walks, try to head back home before you start feeling tired. When you're out there and feeling great is the time to head for home." I smiled. "And, of course, you should take a buddy. Sheila or one of the kids. Why not make it a family project? It'll be good for your new life-style."

He flashed me a rueful look. "You're really out to make me over, aren't you?"

I sat down. "Let's level. In the two and a half weeks you've been here, have you been scared at all?"

"Lots of times."

"For instance . . ."

"Hell, from the minute I first phoned you, and you told me to drop everything and get my ass down here, I was scared. The only reason I was telling you how much work I had and could I delay coming down was I was just testing to find out how serious you were, or really, how serious my condition was. I didn't want to believe it was that bad."

"That happens with every person with chest pains bad enough to call the doctor."

"And then when they stretched me out on the table and attached everything to me but the bathroom sink and kept sticking me for blood samples—yes, I was scared."

"Why?"

"*Why?* You know damn well why! I thought I was going over the edge."

"And did a lot of things that were important suddenly seem less so? The business? The tennis tournament you were missing?"

"Hell, I didn't even think about them."

"Being on the edge has a way of giving you a more basic sense of values. We never know how lucky we are until something threatens to take it all away."

"Well, I sure know now."

"Frank, did you ever see that Noel Coward movie, *The Scoundrel*? Maybe on the late movie on TV?"

"I don't watch TV, outside of sports."

"That figures. Anyway, Noel Coward plays a miserable character who shafts everyone and then dies in a crash. He's heading straight for hell and then gets a second chance. He's put back on earth and told if he can make amends to all the people he's wronged, his bad record will be wiped out and he can start clean. That's who I'm comparing you to."

"Oh, thanks a lot, Doctor. Just who the hell have I shafted?"

"Yourself. All your previous bad health habits have shafted you. But you've got a second chance. Make amends, treat yourself right from now on, and you'll be all right."

He looked at me, frowning. "What are you trying to say, Harold?"

"Frank, *I'm* not out to make you over. You're going to have to do that yourself, and you've got two weeks to lay the foundations of this new person before you start going back to work—two weeks to begin learning to relax and unwind, to enjoy your family and let them enjoy you."

"Let them enjoy me? Am I supposed to do parlor tricks?"

"You don't have to do anything except let them fuss over you."

He winced. "Do I have to get fussed over?"

"What do you think we've been doing to you here for three weeks?"

"Well, this is a hospital."

"Look, for the next week or two, your home is going to be a halfway house."

"A what?"

"Like what they've established for people coming out of institutions where they can learn to adjust to the outside world."

"You mean, for ex-convicts?"

"Not just ex-convicts. People coming out of hospitals need periods of readjustment, too."

"Absolutely, Warden."

I laughed. "Frank, you're still in a state where you could use a little fussing over. A few breakfasts in bed, someone bringing you the paper, that sort of thing. It's important for you to learn to accept and appreciate having things done for you."

He didn't look convinced. Frank was one of that great army of people geared only to give but whose facility for accepting was underdeveloped.

"You know your wife and kids have been through an emotional wringer, too. Don't think they haven't been just as worried as you, maybe more so. Doing things for you now is one way they can show you how much they love you and how glad they are to have you back."

I wasn't prepared for the depth of Frank's reaction. His face went red and he turned away a moment.

"O.K., O.K.," he mumbled. "I'll learn to enjoy. I'll learn to love it."

"Don't go overboard. Just learn to like it. You can get too dependent on being taken care of."

"You mean play invalid the rest of my life."

"Right."

"I won't, don't worry. There's a buyer I used to do business with who had a coronary about four years back. Got out of the hospital and after a month at home his doctor said he was fine. But you know his wife still takes his pulse three times a day plus his blood pressure every morning and night. Does everything but wipe him. Take my word, I won't go overboard."

"Take all the help you can at the beginning, enjoy it, appreciate it, then as you feel yourself getting stronger, less tired, start doing more and more for yourself. No matter how long each new thing takes you to do when you first tackle it, don't let anyone take it over with a 'Here, Dad, let me.' Not once you've started doing things for yourself and feel up to it. The chances are in good time you'll be doing everything you did before you had your coronary."

"Including tennis?"

He *was* persistent. "Yes, including tennis. But learn to also enjoy those walks with Sheila and activity with the kids."

He gave me an answering smile and for once it had no mockery in it. "I will. And, ah, Harold—thank you very much." It was the first note of humility I'd heard from him.

I changed the subject abruptly. "How's the food been?"

"Not bad. Only the portions are so small and they won't give me seconds on anything but water."

"Blame me. It's how I've ordered for you."

He gave me a reproachful look. "No eggs and only skim milk?"

"Frank, how much did you lose since you got in the hospital?"

"About twelve pounds."

"That's about twelve pounds less for your heart to have to nourish or carry around."

Frank approvingly looked down at his noticeably diminished middle. "All those years of tennis didn't do what one coronary did. A heart attack's a great way to lose weight, huh?"

"Yes, if you enjoy Russian Roulette. Try dieting next time. Still, it should really give you a great incentive to stick to a diet."

"You know, I haven't been down to this weight since Sheila and I were married. Unfortunately, she turned out to be a talented cook."

"That's fortunate, not unfortunate. Now she can use those talents on these." I pulled a stapled sheaf of papers out of my pocket and handed it to him.

"Oh, a diet." He scanned it hostilely. "How long do I have to stay on it?"

"Well, you lost twelve pounds in the hospital. How long do you want to keep them off?"

"A lifetime sentence, huh?"

"Your weight is down and all you have to do is keep it down. It's like when driving, you've decelerated to the right speed and now you only need to keep your foot steady on the gas. And you've got someone at home who loves cooking, who can make diet dishes appetizing—you've got it made."

Frank studied the diet sheets intently. "Hey, how come only two or three eggs a week?" All feistiness again.

"You could eat egg whites all day long, they're all protein. But you've got to limit yourself on yolks. They're pure fat."

"But how come so *few* eggs?"

"For the same reason there's so little shellfish on that list, or bacon, or cheeses made from whole milk and cream."

"Aren't they all low-calorie foods? I thought you want people to lose weight, you're supposed to feed them low-calorie foods?"

"There are a lot of low-calorie dishes on that list. Chicken, fish, jack cheese, green vegetables, yellow vegetables, fruit. Low calorie that are also low on cholesterol."

"Oh, that's right, cholesterol, yeah. Doctor, you believe all that stuff about cholesterol?"

"If you're asking me," I said carefully, "whether I believe that a high intake of cholesterol-rich foods may, on occasion, lead to a high level of cholesterol in the bloodstream and that multiplies the chances of a coronary attack, then I must tell you that *most* doctors and dieticians in this country believe that."

"What about you?"

"Shall we say I'm not as positive as some, but I'm not in disagreement with them."

"Cagey, cagey, Doc." He grinned, then shook his head. "The more I read the more confused I get. We need cholesterol, don't we?"

"We couldn't live without it. It helps keep our cells intact, our hair growing, and our skin from drying out; it protects the red blood corpuscles. Most important, it helps the body digest fat."

"Isn't cholesterol a fat?"

I shook my head. "It's greasy and it doesn't dissolve in water, just like fat doesn't. But it's not really fat, although it's found in animal fat. When you eat anything with cholesterol in it, the cholesterol breaks up into microscopic particles. The theory is that a lot of the particles catch onto the artery walls and work their way into the tissue and start forming protrusions that more cholesterol particles cling to. In time the artery passage gets narrower and narrower and if it ever plugs up—"

". . . You've got an arterial occlusion," Frank picked up glibly, "followed immediately by a myocardial infarction."

"Bravo!" I said admiringly.

He looked down at the diet sheets I had given him. "Yeah, you got it all here." He read aloud. " 'All animal fats—lard, suet, salt pork, bacon, meat drippings, marbling on steak, butter, hydrogenated margerine, shortening, etc.—are saturated fat, as is coconut oil. Vegetable oils—olive oil and peanut oil—are unsaturated and contribute no cholesterol to the diet. On the other hand, vegetable oils such as corn oil, soya bean oil, safflower oil, and cottonseed oil are polyunsaturated and have the unique ability to lower the cholesterol count in your bloodstream. For these reasons, it is essential for you to use polyunsaturated oils and margerines in your diet whenever possible.' "

He put down the diet sheet. "So the whole idea is to keep your cholesterol down, right?"

"Right."

"I read where the liver also manufactures cholesterol, a lot of it."

"Oh yes. It can manufacture four or five times as much as you eat."

"Then what's the point of cutting down on cholesterol when your own liver can flood your system with it and there's nothing you can do about that?"

There was a singlemindedness about Frank's questioning that I found interesting.

"There's a lot you can do about it. The liver only manufactures cholesterol to help digest saturated fat. The less animal fat you eat, the less cholesterol your liver will manufacture.

"So a low-cholesterol, high-polyunsaturate diet is what the doctor orders, eh?" He sounded like a trial lawyer.

"It's considered an important factor in lowering heart disease. That's been proven time and again."

"Has it? You know, Harold, I've been reading up on cholesterol and I'd like to read you something on it." He picked up a book from the night table. *The Cholesterol Controversy* by Edward R. Pinkney, M.D. and Cathey

Pinckney. "Now listen to this, Doc." He was practically Mr. District Attorney as he opened it to a carefully marked page. " 'During the past two decades, the "average" American has increased his consumption of polyunsaturates to three times the quantity that was eaten back in the 1940s. At the same time he has reduced his intake of dairy foods, eggs, beef, and pork no less than half. And with all this, the heart disease rate has climbed almost parallel to the rise of polyunsaturates in the diet. Certainly if polyunsaturates really did work as claimed . . . we should have had some reduction in heart attacks. But instead all forms of heart disease have actually skyrocketed.' "

He closed the book and looked at me. "Think maybe those figures are fake?"

"Oh, I'm perfectly willing to accept them."

"Then you accept the fact that polyunsaturates don't work."

"Of course I don't."

"But you just said you accept what I read you—the more polyunsaturates in the diet the last twenty years, the more heart disease has skyrocketed."

"Frank, in the last twenty years the number of psychiatrists has multiplied. So has the number of mentally ill people. The number of police has zoomed. So has the amount of crime. Does that mean we should give up psychiatrists and police? Or does that mean that conditions in society, over which police and psychiatrists have no control, have produced more and more disturbed minds and more and more crime? While society tries to grapple with the basic problems, psychiatrists and police keep them from growing worse."

"Are you saying that without low-cholesterol diets, there'd be more heart disease?"

"Probably. Look at the evidence. You feed animals like

rabbits, monkeys, pigeons excess cholesterol they get coronary disease . . ."

"Yeah, I read about those experiments. They feed them pure cholesterol. I mean like more than a hundred times what people eat, even people who eat a lot of cholesterol. Wouldn't you say they're loading the dice?"

"Well, if I told you that those rabbits, pigeons, et cetera developed atherosclerosis in three to sixteen months, whereas people who ingest cholesterol as a small fraction of their diet take forty or fifty years to develop a coronary condition, wouldn't you say that kind of evens it out?"

Frank shrugged. "Hell, who cares about a pigeon's heart trouble. Let's talk about people."

"Right, let's talk about people. Some years ago, there was an international medical study of some ten thousand men from several different countries, including the U.S., for a period of ten years. They found that the higher the cholesterol level in the normal diet of the country studied, the higher the rate of coronary thrombosis among the male population."

"Where do we stand?"

"We were second highest. Finland was first. They eat more animal fat, pro rata, than we do. The Japanese, who have the lowest cholesterol level in their diet, have the lowest coronary rate."

Frank's lip curled. "In my business we use statistics, too. What's the trend in slacks going to be next year in Dallas or Toronto or Tokyo? Or will dresses outsell suits in Kansas City, depending on the price of wheat or cattle? So I know how you can hook numbers together like that. The amount of cholesterol in a diet in a country as against the rise in coronaries. You could find that it might hook up even better with the amount of business failures in each country or the number of automobile accidents or the number of blondes. Statistical comparatives are tricky things."

I couldn't help laughing. "O.K., Frank, you're the doctor. How about this one? In Framingham, Massachusetts, a group of healthy respected scientists have been performing a long-term epidemiological study on thousands of people. They have been analyzing a number of coronary risk factors such as blood pressure, cholesterol level, smoking habits, EKG abnormalities, and sugar intolerance in persons of both sexes in all age groups. We can now refer to a table and forecast a patient's statistical chances of having coronary problem if we know all things about him."

"Sounds like a ouija board."

"No, it's more like an insurance company's actuarial table."

"O.K., what'd they find out?"

"Disregarding other factors, the forecast is that men with high cholesterol levels are three times likelier to have heart disease than men with low cholesterol readings. And it's been working out that way with great accuracy."

Frank glared at the diet sheet.

"So it comes to this," I went on, "you can follow a fat-controlled, low-cholesterol diet zealously and still have a heart attack, just as a motorist can follow all the rules in the book and still not be able to avoid an accident. But just because the model driver sometimes gets hit doesn't give the rest of us dispensation to forget the rules. You follow a diet designed to lower blood cholesterol levels and the chances are you're helping yourself."

Frank read from the diet sheet. " 'No more than sixteen ounces of beef, pork, or lamb per week. Fish, five times a week.' Did you think this list up?"

"With some help from the Bureau of Nutrition of the New York City Health Department of 1957."

"You weren't practicing medicine in New York in 1957, were you?"

"No, but that was the year the New York Health Department formed an 'anticoronary club' to find out if a fat-restricted diet could reduce the level of cholesterol in the blood and whether that would reduce the incidence of coronary disease. The Bureau of Nutrition worked out a diet in which animal fats and unsaturated fat products were balanced. Less meat, more fish sort of thing. Like the diet you're holding in your hand."

"What happened with the club?"

"About nine hundred men between the ages of forty and fifty-nine joined. Later they formed another club, a sort of control group of men of about the same age span and the same health level. The nine-hundred-member anticoronary club went on the diet. The control group ate what they had been eating all along."

"What happened?"

"In six months, the members of the anticoronary club all lost weight. That was good because obesity is considered by many doctors as another coronary risk factor. But more importantly, their cholesterol levels all went down. The higher the level a man had, the greater the drop."

"What about coronaries?"

"At the end of eight years, they took the first survey. There were two-thirds less coronaries in the anticoronary club than there were in the control group. More than sixty percent less."

"Say, that's real good."

"Let's say it's not bad. Lowering cholesterol levels is no cure-all, but this study suggests that a change of diet can be helpful."

Frank shook his head. "Harold, I can't figure you out.

One minute, you're beating the drum for your cholesterol theory, next minute you're putting it down."

"I'm not putting it down. I'm putting it in its proper place. Some people can subsist on diets high in cholesterol without any increase in the percentage of cholesterol in their blood. Take the people of Roseta, a small town in Pennsylvania. The population is mostly Italian. Some twenty or so years ago, it was noted that the town had an exceptionally low rate of coronary disease. A survey was taken and it was discovered that the diet of the people of Roseta was exceptionally high in cholesterol, but there was an uncommonly low percentage in their blood. A diet high in cholesterol yet very few cases of coronary disease. How would you account for that?"

"Let me see. Did they take life easy?"

"Exactly. They were more relaxed. There was very little stress. Stress, anxiety, constant worry, constant fear, apprehension keep the heartbeat going faster. Like a car motor that's always racing. It wears out faster. Any small flaws in it enlarge; and contribute to the breakdown. In Roseta, however, there was very little stress. It was almost a rural atmosphere. Everyone at work walked home for lunch. Every family had a garden, raised their own vegetables. So even though they ate a lot of pasta, spaghetti, and gravy, the relaxed quality of life and possibly their heriditary pattern seem to have counterbalanced the high-cholesterol meals. Then factories started moving into Roseta, there was an industrial boom. The relaxed atmosphere disappeared and with it the exceptionally low coronary rate. Today, Roseta has as many heart patients in the county hospitals as does every other town in the county."

"So what you're saying is that stress is the villain, not cholesterol."

"When it comes to coronary disease, there's not just one villain. When you start living under stress a higher amount of cholesterol may start to show up in the bloodstream, and there's more danger of coronary arteries clogging up with cholesterol and fatty deposits. Stress is a villain, so is cholesterol, so is a bad family history, so is heridity, and there are others, too."

"Being overweight?"

"Yes. The more weight you put on, the harder your heart has to work to carry it around. If you take someone who lives under high pressure all the time . . ."

"Stress."

"Right, and who's grossly overweight and who eats a high-cholesterol diet, well, if they get a coronary, which factor are you going to attribute it to? It's all the factors. But which one is more important in causing the heart trouble can vary from person to person."

"You keep telling me about regular exercise, that's another villain. Or is that the same as losing weight?"

"No, it's a separate factor. A man could be underweight and yet so flabby from sitting around that his heart muscles could be weak. He would not be fit, from a cardiovascular point of view. Losing weight is to give the heart less work. Exercising is to strengthen the heart."

"How about sex?"

I laughed as I shook my head. "Frank, are you sure you just don't have sex on the brain?"

He winked at me. "I'm still waiting for the sex talk you're supposed to give me. How about morale as a factor?"

"Morale is the great all around factor for any illness, but it's not specific for heart disease, like, let us say, giving up cigarettes. . ."

Frank looked unhappy. Prior to his coronary, I had rarely

seen him without a cigarette, except when he was on a tennis court.

"I read that one of those blue-ribbon committees put together by the Surgeon General said that smoking *doesn't* cause coronary heart disease."

"Slight misquote, Frank. What they said was that even though male cigarette smokers have a higher rate of coronary disease than do nonsmokers, they won't quite go as far as to say smoking is the cause."

"So there you are!" Frank said triumphantly.

"There may be a question about whether or not it is the cause of coronary disease, but there's no question at all about the association of smoking to the development of coronary artery disease. Research shows heavy cigarette smokers—'heavy' means ten or more cigarettes a day—are about three times as vulnerable as nonsmokers to coronary disease. Interestingly, pipe and cigar smokers are about as immune as nonsmokers—probably because they don't inhale. It appears that nicotine narrows the coronary blood vessels and produces changes in the bloodstream that predispose cigarette smokers to heart attacks."

"Everything you say about cigarette smoking starts with 'it appears' or 'it seems,'" Frank said tartly.

"That's the way scientists talk about anything that isn't absolutely proven, that's still in the test tube stage. You've got to talk carefully when you're investigating a habit of tens of millions of people."

"O.K., what about the Japanese?"

"What about them?"

"They smoke as much as we do. Don't tell me they don't. I've done business in Tokyo. I know."

"They do smoke as much as we do."

"And they have much fewer coronary cases than we do, both heavy cigarette smokers and nonsmokers, right?"

"Yes."

"O.K. How come?"

"We're not sure."

Frank grinned. "Another way of saying you don't know, isn't it?"

"There are a lot of things we don't know. The Masai tribe in Kenya lives on the milk and blood of their cattle, and they ingest huge amounts of cholesterol. But there's no heart disease among the Masai. Maybe it's because they're a vigorous outdoor people. No obesity. Lots of exercise. On the other hand, the northern Finnish people do a great deal of exercise—skiing, outdoor work, sports. But they also eat a high cholesterol diet. Not as high as the Masai but the highest in Europe. They also have the highest coronary disease rate in Europe."

"What's that got to do with smoking?"

"Frank, a coronary isn't a cold in the head. You get a cold from a single cause, a virus. You cure it by staying warm and resting. A coronary has multiple causes. The risk factors such as high blood pressure, cholesterol, overweight, lack of exercise, cigarette smoking—all in different combinations in different environments and situations—can work differently."

"I'm still asking—"

"Yes, about the Japanese. The Japanese smoke like furnaces and yet they are the industrialized people least susceptible to heart disease. Yet let them settle in the U.S. and in a short time their coronary rate is indistinguishable from Caucasians here."

"Maybe it's the change of diet."

"Maybe. Forget what all the possible reasons may be,

Frank. My advice is to cut out all cigarette smoking. Period."

"O.K., O.K.," he said peevishly. "I'll take up marijuana."

I threw up my hands in mock despair. "Here I try to turn you toward a healthier second life, and first you're playing the ponies and now you're smoking pot!"

"Well, you're cutting me off cigarettes. What do you expect? There's no nicotine in grass, is there?"

"No, but they've been doing research . . ."

"Here we go," he sighed. "The test tube stuff. It appears that it seems that maybe . . ."

"Marijuana doesn't have any nicotine in it, but it produces carbon monoxide, which has enormous affinity for hemoglobin. Hemoglobin carries oxygen to the lungs. When you smoke grass, carbon monoxide is sucked into the lungs and displaces the oxygen that would normally be carried by the hemoglobin to the cells."

"So?"

"So your blood is less oxygenated and that means your ability to sustain exercise is curtailed. You're getting less oxygen to burn, so you get tired in half the time. If you were an angina patient doing exercise, your heart would start to hurt from the workout a lot sooner."

"I wasn't planning to smoke pot and exercise at the same time."

"I'm just giving you the facts, Frank. I admit there hasn't been enough research done on cannibas to draw definite conclusions. But except the relaxing effect it may have on many people, it doesn't do anybody any good."

"You sure are a lot of fun today, Doc."

At that moment, the door opened and a brunette vision in a chic outfit walked into the room. On seeing me, she stopped.

"Oh, I'm sorry," she faltered, "I thought you were alone."

"Oh, Melanie, this is my doctor . . ." Frank responded with alacrity. "Doctor . . . um . . ."

"Karpman," I said.

"Yeah. Doctor, this is Melanie Peters, one of the models at my place, just dropped in to see me."

"How do you do, Doctor." She turned her large blue eyes on Frank. "I didn't know you had other visitors. I guess I'd better go."

"No, no," Frank said. "Dr. Karpman took longer than usual. He's about finished I think, aren't you . . . ?"

"No," I replied.

I enjoyed Frank's look of surprise. "Oh? Ah, O.K. Ah, Melanie, why don't you wait outside for a while?"

"All right," she said reluctantly. "I hope I won't have to wait too long, I'd hate to be late for work. What would I tell the boss?" She giggled and winked at her boss on the bed, then left.

Frank looked embarrassed.

"Frank," I said, "you've been asking me when I'm going to give you your sex talk."

"Yeah."

"Well, how about right now?"

11. Heavy Traffic on a Jammed Street

"How long do the pains go on?"

"Like I said on the phone, Doctor—over a year." Thornhill had the truculent speech of an old New York City cop, which, it turned out, he had been for thirty years.

"No, I mean how long do they last each time they happen?"

"Ohhhhh." Thornhill drew it out to suggest that I hadn't framed the question clearly, not that he had misunderstood. His wife must often find him irritating, it occurred to me. "About half a minute," he said.

"Half a minute. And you get them walking up steps."

"In my apartment house. Lots of times I come home, that elevator is tied up above the tenth floor. You press that button, you got a long while to wait."

"So you walk up the stairs."

"Why not? Our place is only on the sixth floor. But

damned if every time I walk up I don't get these squeezing, burning pains in my chest."

"Do you get them anywhere besides your chest?"

"Sometimes they grab me around the Adam's apple, sometimes the back of my neck, my left arm, even my teeth. I got to stop before they go away. Weekends, when I'm in no hurry, it's easier getting up the stairs, unless I'm carrying groceries."

"When you get the pains, do you take the elevator?"

"Yeah. And by the time I'm in the apartment I feel fine."

"Do you get those chest pains on other occasions besides when you're climbing stairs?"

"Well, last summer, the wife and I were on a vacation up in the San Gabriel Mountains. I'd get chest pains sometimes walking uphill."

"Was it cold and windy up there?"

"Sometimes."

"What do you do for exercise generally, Mr. Thornhill?"

"Exercise?" He chortled, jowels rippling. He had a chin like a punching bag, and a paunch to match. "What do you think my job is, if not exercise?" I looked at his chart. He was head of security for a discount department store. "On my feet all day, going up and down from floor to floor!"

"Your store has elevators, doesn't it?"

"Never use them. Unless I'm tailing shoplifters."

"What about escalators?"

"Sure. But I don't stand still on 'em. I move my tail."

"Do you ever use the stairs?"

"Sometimes."

"How often?"

"Now and then."

"How often is now and then?"

He flushed. "Hey, what's this—the third degree?"

I laughed. "Now, would I give an old cop the third degree? Look, you told me every time you walk up the stairs of your apartment house, you get chest pains. If that means you're overexerting by walking up those stairs, then I have a good idea of what your problem is. But when you tell me that you're on your feet all day on your job and you go up and down from floor to floor and you don't get chest pains, then *I've* got the problem. Why should you get chest pains climbing the apartment stairs and not the store stairs?"

Now it was difficult to tell if Thornhill's face was flushed from irritation or embarrassment.

"Well, my apartment is six floors up, but the store's only two floors. Maybe I'm not doing much climbing at work. I guess I must use the staircase only one or two times a month. Rest of the time I use the escalator. You climb three steps on an escalator and you're on the next floor."

"What about being on your feet all day?"

He looked even more sheepish. "Well, not really all day. I got an office and a couch."

Thornhill wasn't the first patient I've had whose initial description of himself broke down under questioning.

"But there's nothing the matter with my heart," he said defiantly. "My old lady was after me to see a doctor. So I went to the company clinic, took an EKG. Got a clean bill of health. Didn't stop my old lady. 'You still get those chest pains, go see a heart doctor!' She can be a pain too, and not in the chest." He chuckled.

"At least it got you to come in to see me. What kind of an electrocardiograph was it, Mr. Thornhill?"

"What do you mean what kind?"

"Well, were you lying down and resting when you took it?"

"Yeah. You mean there are other kinds?"

"Oh, yes. Now, tell me—do you and your wife argue a lot?"

"I never argue," he said piously, "but sometimes she drives me into sounding off."

"And when you sound off, do you get those chest pains?"

He paused to think. "Yeah, but never for more'n a couple of minutes."

"Once you feel them do you stop sounding off?"

"Yeah."

"And do the pains subside?"

"Oh, yes. In about three minutes."

"Mr. Thornhill, have you ever had a chest injury or broken any bones in, say, the last ten years?"

"Nope. I fractured an ankle once chasing a purse snatcher who scored off an old woman. Caught the son of a bitch, too. That was nineteen years ago."

I moved on to his family history. Were any blood relatives chronically ill? What about deceased relatives? What had they died of? I wanted to find out if there was a family history of cardiovascular disease or hypertension. I then took his own medical history. Had he had any operations, serious illnesses, injuries? What were his sleeping patterns, work patterns, smoking habits? How many cups of coffee or tea did he consume a day? Did he use any drugs? Aspirin? Heroin? ("Hell, no!" he exploded—so fiercely I was glad the room was sound-proofed.) Had he had any trouble with his eyes, ears, nose, throat, mouth, head?

"Well, that's that," I finally said.

He heaved a great sigh of relief. "About time! I been cross-examined by some of the best trial lawyers in New York in my time. You press pretty good yourself."

"I'm only doing the sort of thing someone investigating crime does—getting all the evidence together and sifting through it to find the guilty party." I stood up. "Now let's go into the examining room."

Thornhill looked thunderstruck. "The examining room?"

"Yes, I want to check you over, take some tests—"

"Mother of Jesus! You mean after all the questions you can't tell me why I'm getting those pains?"

"I think I can, Mr. Thornhill, but I have to corroborate my diagnosis in the examining room. Like when you were a policeman. A crime is committed, someone comes up and confesses he did it, and that's fine, but you want some hard evidence before you take him in, don't you?"

"Doc, if you'd been on the force as long as I was, you'd know a killer from a kook before he opened his mouth."

"I'm sure. But still, you can't bring a confessed killer before a judge without evidence, can you?"

Thornhill sighed with the long-suffering tolerance of a cop for a civilian. "O.K., Doc, what did I confess to?"

"In a minute I'll be happy to tell you."

In the examining room, I inspected every nook and cranny of Thornhill's body. I looked at the eyes, observing the pupils and their reaction to light. Using an ophthalmoscope I looked in the back of the eye, the only place in the body where the arteries and veins can be usually inspected without surgery. I checked the ears, nose, and throat, and then the neck, chest, lungs, heart, abdomen, genitalia, extremities, and neurological system. I examined the rectum to be sure his prostate was not enlarged or irregular. Among other things I wanted to make sure his symptoms weren't connected to some ailment coming from someplace other than the heart.

I finally told him to put his clothes on and left the room

briefly to check another patient. When I returned, he was dressed—and anxious. "Well?"

"Well, tomorrow we take tests."

His jaw dropped. "What the hell was happening today?"

"The first part of a thorough medical checkup. Tomorrow morning, we'll concentrate on your cardiovascular system. The secretary will give you an appointment. Incidentally, don't eat anything after midnight tonight. It might affect some of the tests."

"What about beer?"

"Only until midnight," I said. "After that, nothing."

He sighed. "My old lady'll really think I'm sick."

Next morning, I had blood specimens and a urine sample collected, and had x-rays taken of his chest and abdomen.

"Now," I told him, "we're going to get a cardiogram."

"But I told you I've had one already! And I passed, too!"

"You had the *resting* electrocardiogram," I said. "We'll repeat that so that we'll be certain what your heart waves are like under resting conditions. Then we'll take it in the sitting and standing positions after you've been breathing deeply and then while you're holding your breath. The grand finale will be the treadmill exercise stress test."

Thornhill stripped to the waist in our cardiac stress laboratory. His hairy chest revealed a shaved area the size of a silver dollar on each side of his chest. "See?" he said pointing to them, "I told you I had an EKG."

"Well, it saves me the job of shaving you," said Carol, the EKG technician.

She applied electrodes and recorded the various cardiograms of him, which formed the baseline records. Thornhill was then asked to stand on the treadmill. He stood self-consciously holding his stomach in, wires dangling from his chest, which would connect with the cardioscope that would monitor his heart.

"The treadmill will start slowly, a little under two miles an hour, and the incline will at first be slight, only about a ten percent grade. Then every three minutes we'll increase both the speed and the pitch of the treadmill. Now, the important thing is if you feel any pain or pressure—in your chest, arms, neck, shoulders, back, or anywhere else—you must tell me immediately. I may want to stop the test and get the EKG reading at that moment. It's also absolutely vital that you let me know *immediately* if you have even the slightest pain. Got that?"

"Got it," he grunted. "Let's go."

The treadmill started at the easy rate of 1.7 miles per hour, and he walked easily at a steady pace. "Reminds me of a beat I had in Brooklyn Heights a long time back," he said. "Just as steep and just as boring."

"Mr. Thornhill," Carol cautioned, "it would be a good idea not to do any talking because it'll tire you and throw off the test."

At the end of the first three minutes his heart had accelerated from 88 beats per minute to 135, but the oscilloscope indicated no evidence of cardiac abnormalities or arrhythmias. I told Thornhill we would raise the incline to 12 percent and the speed to 2.5 miles per hour.

In two more minutes he was breathing more heavily. Watching the oscilloscope, I noticed that certain EKG changes were occurring which strongly suggested myocardial ischemia, an inadequate blood flow through the coronary arteries. However, no abnormal rhythms of the heart were evident yet.

"Getting tougher, Doctor," he panted.

"How do you mean?" I asked.

"Beginning to get a little pressure. In the chest," he gasped.

"O.K., we'll stop now."

I stopped the treadmill and Carol then gave Thornhill a brief standing cardiogram, followed by a full resting cardiogram each minute for the next ten minutes. The evidence of myocardial ischemia was observable in the first six tracings. The treadmill study had confirmed my clinical impression.

"Now I can tell you without question," I told him later in my office, "the pains you've been feeling are called anginal pains. All the tests point to a condition known as angina pectoris."

"Angina . . . me? What the hell is that?"

"Angina pectoris means 'pain in the chest.' You've got all the classic symptoms—the burning, squeezing feeling in the chest. Sometimes it radiates to the neck, to the jaw, to the shoulder and arms. In fact, much of the time it goes to the left shoulder and arm, even to the elbow or fingers. Sometimes it's to the pit of the stomach. Generally, the pain comes from overexerting yourself in an activity you're not used to doing any more, or maybe never were, such as climbing stairs, climbing a hill, running. Sometimes it comes from being cold or being hit by a chill wind or from being very angry."

"Does it have anything to do with the heart?"

"I'm afraid it does. As we get older, we tend to accumulate fat deposits on the inside walls of our coronary arteries, the ones that supply blood to the heart. The deposits become like grease inside a pipe, and it gets harder for the blood to flow through."

"Is that what's called artero, arterio . . . ?"

"Arteriosclerosis?"

"Yeah."

"In a way of speaking. Arteriosclerosis means a hardening of the arteries. Atherosclerosis is a form of arteriosclerosis in which fat and cholesterol deposits accumulate inside coronary arteries."

Thornhill pulled a pencil and thick pad from his back pocket. "Spell that."

I did and then continued. "The passageways inside the sections of the coronary arteries affected keep getting narrower, but still enough blood can get through to supply oxygen and food to heart tissues to keep the heart functioning under normal conditions. But when you really exert yourself—as when you're walking upstairs or when you're quarreling or you're very cold—you need a lot more energy faster, which means your tissues need oxygen faster."

Thornhill jotted in his notebook with grim concentration. I paused. He looked up expectantly.

"Do you always write things down?" I asked.

He looked surprised. "It's a cop habit. You mind?"

"Oh, no. But I keep getting this funny feeling you're giving me a ticket."

He studied me a full three seconds before a grin broke out on the square face. He started to put the pad back into his pocket.

"No, no, it's O.K. to take notes. A doctor's got to learn to adjust, too." Thornhill resumed jotting.

"O.K.," I went on, "with the fat deposits narrowing them, the coronary arteries can allow only a thin stream of blood through. So if the heart muscle needs more blood and the narrowed coronary arteries can't increase the flow, you get a warning signal, chest pains, and you have to stop doing what you're doing—walking upstairs or whatever."

Thornhill frowned. "Well, how come the cardiogram at the store clinic showed my ticker doing just fine?"

"Look at it this way. Say you're directing traffic on a crosstown street—say Forty-second Street in New York. It's a wide street normally, right? But let's say it's got parked cars lining both sides, so now it's lost two lanes. However, since it's early in the afternoon and there are not too many cars, traffic is running smoothly. That's what it's like for someone with coronary atherosclerosis under normal circumstances. Coronary arteries may be narrowed here and there, but traffic is running smoothly."

"Then comes rush hour," Thornhill said, getting the idea.

"Exactly. Thousands of more cars trying to get through streets already narrowed by cars parked on both sides. It becomes a real jam. To someone with angina pectoris, things like overexertion, anger, or sudden chill are like heavy traffic on a jammed street. And none of that shows up when you take a resting cardiogram. When a person's flat on his back, even a diseased heart often registers as normal. That's why I put you on the treadmill."

Thornhill continued scribbling.

"Now if you start getting cars *double*-parked," I went on, "hardly any traffic's going to get through on that street, right? The whole thing gets blocked. That constriction is called a coronary occlusion. And the result of that is that you'd be having a myocardial infarction—fancy name for a heart attack."

"So that's why you stopped the treadmill test right away," Thornhill said. "I could of had a heart attack on that thing just like that!"

"Mr. Thornhill, anyone can have a heart attack anywhere anytime. Angina is a warning. It says your chances are greater if you don't do something about it."

"Well, what am I supposed to do?"

"You've done it already."

"Yeah?"

"You've come to a doctor, O.K.? So now we can start reducing the chances of a heart attack."

"How?"

"If you've got to have a heart condition, angina is the best kind. So, if you have an attack of angina and stop what you're doing right then and there—cool your temper, get in out of the cold, whatever—the chest and neck pain will usually stop in a matter of minutes. An angina pain doesn't do the heart any harm. It's not like a coronary occlusion. There the blood supply is cut off and the muscle is injured."

"Hey, but you just told me you can go right from an angina condition into a heart attack."

"Yes, but the pains are a warning. They're telling you to cut down on your stresses and strains. They're saying improve your way of living so you won't go to something worse. Angina pectoris in fact, is one of those ailments whose pain we can usually treat very effectively with drugs." He frowned. "Nothing addictive," I added. "These are just drugs to prevent the pain from coming on. Or if they do come on, to eliminate them quickly."

"You mean all you got to do is take it and the pain stops?"

"That's right. They're called nitroglycerin. When you feel a chest pain, put a nitroglycerin tablet under your tongue. It'll dissolve quickly, and in a matter of seconds it'll go through your system and the pain will be gone. The effect lasts only a few minutes, but by that time, presumably, you've stopped doing whatever brought on the attack. You can also take one to ward off pain. Like when you know you have to walk upstairs rapidly. Take it beforehand and you won't feel any pain the entire way up. Nitroglycerin expands the coronary arteries to let extra blood flow into your heart arteries."

Thornhill grinned. "Forty-second Street getting wider during the rush hour. The dream of Times Square Precinct." Then he frowned. "Wait a minute. Is this nitroglycerin the same as in dynamite?"

"Yes, but there's absolutely no danger of being blown up. There's only a small amount in each tablet. It's a safe medication. Some people have taken as many as twenty or thirty a day.

Thornhill wagged his head. "How about that. Same stuff that can kill people can cure 'em."

True enough. And there are similar paradoxes with other drugs. Curare is used to reduce hypertension, yet it is derived from a root used by South American Indians on the tips of their arrows as a powerful, deadly poison. But to a cardiologist nitroglycerin is particularly important. Once when there was a series of fatal and near-fatal cases of coronary insufficiency in employees of a Midwestern munitions factory, an associate and I were asked to help investigate it. The factory manufactured a nitroglycerin-cellulose mixture for solid rocket propellant. Most acute heart episodes took place on Sunday night or Monday morning and none of the victims had a history of heart ailments, high blood pressure, diabetes, or other such predisposing factors. Indeed, autopsies showed those who died suddenly had coronary blood vessels that were relatively normal and healthy. All were from small towns or rural areas within miles of the plant.

I was amazed to find that, even in 1970, explosives were made much the same way they were before World War I—in small, concrete huts encased in logs, debris, and dirt, open to the sky like Indian tents. No more than eight workers were allowed in any one hut at once. And the huts were widely separated in case of an accident.

At the time we were called in, eight female and one male employees, in a work force of 200, had developed signs of coronary insufficiency, four fatally.

Interestingly, a sort of folklore preventative measure had sprung up among the employees. On Friday night, at the end of the work week, several employees would take small vials of the powdered nitroglycerin home. On Saturday and Sunday mornings they would dust themselves with the powder, or moisten it into a paste and rub it over their bodies. And on Saturday and Sunday nights, they would shower off the residue—just as they showered at the end of every work day at the plant. None of those who took this weekend "fix" suffered from what was known as Monday Morning Disease—that is, recurrent and severe anginal pains—though none had a scientific explanation for the ritual.

In our research, we found that Monday Morning Disease had been described since the early 1900s in European and American munitions factories. The villain, it developed, was nitroglycerin. Though the munitions company provided employees with protective rubber gloves, aprons, work clothes, and an excellent ventilation system, the nitroglycerin particles being manufactured were so fine that much would seep through the clothes onto the skin. This would be absorbed into the circulatory system, causing the arteries to expand. At the end of the work day, employees had showered off the excess powder and gone home. But unless there was nitroglycerin on the skin being absorbed into the system, their coronary arteries would slowly constrict—until next morning when they went back to work, and new dust on the skins would start their arteries expanding again.

By itself, this regular constriction-dilation of their arteries did no harm. However, because of the weekend break in the expand-contract rhythm, and because certain workers were peculiarly sensitive, their arteries got narrower than usual on Saturdays and Sundays. By Monday the coronary arteries would constrict so tightly that no blood could get through, and they suffered anginal pains, heart attacks, and even death. Thus, the folk remedy of rubbing nitroglycerin powder on the skin on weekends turned out to be the best preventative.

"Now," I told Thornhill, as I wrote out the prescriptions, "there are two kinds of drugs that will do you good. First, of course, are nitroglycerin tablets. Carry them with you at all times, and when you feel the slightest angina twinge—or do something you think may give you angina pain—put one under your tongue to dissolve."

"Doctor," Thornhill interrupted, "is nitroglycerin, ah, you know, habit forming?"

"No," I smiled. "Nor is the other pill I'm prescribing."

"What's that pill?"

"It's a long-acting coronary artery dilator. It will keep your arteries enlarged for longer periods of time than a nitro tablet will. Hopefully, it will also reduce your need for nitroglycerin."

Thornhill stopped scratching in his book and put it away. "Know what, Doctor? I feel better now that I really know what's going on—what the cause of the pain really is."

"Good," I said. "Then you should know there's something else interesting about angina—it's susceptible to how relaxed the patient is. If you have confidence in your doctor's ability to handle your case, your angina pains will probably decrease in frequency. They've tested people with angina pectoris by giving them a placebo—a fake pill with no medical value—instead of a nitro tablet, and have found that the angina pains will disappear in some patients if they think they're taking a nitroglycerin.

I handed Thornhill the prescriptions.

"Say, maybe you oughta give me the fake pills," he said. "Bet they'd cost a lot less."

"Bet they would." I grinned. "But they wouldn't work on you now. You know too much. If you want to avoid taking pills or at least cut down on them, go to a warm climate. The warmer it is, the less angina pain."

"I'll keep it in mind for our next vacation." Thornhill carefully folded the prescriptions and put them in his wallet.

"A couple more things," I said. "First, I want you to cut down on your calories. Bring your weight down to the ideal level for your height and bone structure. Second, anytime you're doing something that gives you even a twinge in your chest area, quit immediately—no overexertion. Stay out of drafts and dress warmly for cold weather. A third thing. Exercise regularly, at least three times a week."

"Hold it right there," Thornhill said. "First you said no overexertion, then you said exercise."

"Right. Exercise until you feel that first twinge in the chest, then quit. As you exercise, as you diet, as you protect yourself, your heart muscle will get stronger and require less added energy for exertions. As you lose weight, your heart has less pumping to do, even under normal circumstances. Angina pectoris is improvable."

"Improvable, eh, Doc, I'm the kind of guy who likes his food, beer, and comfort, but I think I can lick this angina."

"How about yelling back at your wife?"

He grinned. "Listen, when I was a patrolman we used the

buddy system on the beat. Did a better job, too, because it was our beat. Well, on this, the old lady and I can be buddies, too."

He started to leave the office, then turned. "Hey. What you said about writing in a pad was like a cop giving you a ticket?"

"Yes?"

"Well, funny thing. You know, you're like the cop who tore up a ticket and said, 'O.K., you're getting another chance.'"

I liked that.

12. The Sex Commandment

"Now? You want to talk about sex *now?*" Frank's surprise bordered on shock. He sat up and pulled down primly on his pajama top as though it were the jacket of a business suit. "Why now?"

"Why not now?" I pulled a chair toward the bed and sat down. "You're going home to your wife soon, you've brought up the subject a few times—"

"Doctor, does it have anything to do with . . . ?" He nodded at the door that his well-endowed employee had just closed behind her. "You don't think for a minute that she and I . . ."

"Frank, it must be in your mind, not mine. I'm your doctor, not your rabbi. My interest in your sex life is medical, not moral. I've just had the feeling lately that you've got questions about sex, and now's as good a time as any to discuss it."

He got up from the bed and paced the narrow room, avoiding looking at me. "I can't think of anything. I mean, you know, springing it on me like this . . ." He gave the door a fleeting look, then his face lit up. "Hey, aren't there books on sex for people who've had a heart attack?"

"You've got one right in that pile." I indicated the books on his night table. "Myron Benton's *Heart and Sex*. In fact, didn't you quote from it the other day about how squeamish so many doctors are about discussing sex with their patients?"

He nodded impatiently. "Yeah, I skimmed through it. I'll read it carefully and that should take care of things, O.K.?"

"O.K. Well, if you don't have any questions . . ."

"No, I don't." He stood next to my chair as though anxious to escort me to the door.

"In that case, *I* have one," I said, "and I hope you'll answer me frankly."

He sagged with exasperation. "What is it?"

"Frank, do you—?"

"No, I don't. I'm a happily married man and I don't play around."

"O.K., now let me—"

"Melanie just happens to be nice enough to visit her boss in the hospital. Does that answer your question, Doctor?"

"I haven't had a chance to ask it."

"Oh, I'm sorry."

"The question I want to ask is, has sex been more on your mind these last few days since you've been up and around?"

He gave a laugh, which he tried to make ribald. "Well, what do you think, Doc?"

"What sort of thoughts have you been having?"

He shrugged. "You know. The usual thing. Being in the

hay, that sort of thing." He grinned. "You want me to draw you some pictures?"

"Is that the only kind of thoughts?"

He looked at me almost with indignation. "What other kinds of thoughts would you expect me to have . . . about sex?"

"Frank, I told you I'm not a squeamish doctor. Are you a squeamish patient? It's just as unfortunate for the patient who can't level with the doctor as it is for the doctor who can't lay it on the line with the patient."

Frank was silent a moment. He sat down on the bed. "O.K., Doc," he blurted out, "I've been thinking about sex all the time these past two days and I'm scared shitless. I guess that surprises you."

There was no sarcasm.

"No, it doesn't, Frank. It would have surprised me if you hadn't felt like that." Then I added lightly, "But you're wrong about one thing. Your mental state hasn't affected your bowel movement, which happens to be excellent—one reason your recovery has been so good. Straining at your stool is a strain on your heart, you know."

Frank brooded a moment then he said, "If straining at the bowel can be such a strain on the heart, what about sex? Isn't that one of the greatest strains of all?"

"No, sex really isn't that much of a strain. For a middle-aged patient who's had a heart attack, during sexual climax the heartbeat averages 117 beats per minute. But it can go as high as 144 beats per minute—about like the energy expenditure of climbing a flight of stairs. The blood pressure can also go up somewhat."

"You're telling me to go back to it? Take such a chance?"

"You'll be going back to everything you've done before your heart attack, but you'll go back in better shape. As you develop your physical stamina and recondition your body, a normal sex life will be absolutely no threat to your heart. In fact, it will be vital to your complete recovery."

"My sex life?"

"The sex act is a physical one, isn't it? When it's called an indoor sport, there's more truth than humor in that."

He didn't even smile at that one. "But you just told me what a terrible strain on the heart the climax is. Heart beating fast, blood pressure shooting up . . ."

"But that all happens during the orgasm, and how long does that last? Eight seconds? Ten seconds?"

"Look, you can blow out a tire in less than *one* second."

"If the tire is in good shape, it can take all kinds of stresses and strains. That's the shape you have to get back to before you start."

"How will we know when I'm a good tire again?"

"It's not that big a deal. Most sports require much more and much longer effort than an orgasm requires. A few years ago, seven men who had had serious coronaries, most of them worse than yours, entered the Boston Marathon— twenty-six miles over hill and dale. A lot of trained athletes dropped along the way in that race, but all seven ex-cardiacs finished in good shape. They'd been training for three years under their cardiologist's supervision. He had started them off with short, leisurely walks, then longer walks, then a little jogging, then more jogging. In three years he had gradually worked them up to full participation in a sport that takes a lot more out of a man than an orgasm."

Frank gave me a look of mock surprise. "It's going to take me three years of training before I can have an orgasm?"

I laughed. When Frank started being funny, it meant his anxieties were receding. "Sex is a very short sprint, not a marathon. But the principle is the same. You start slowly and work your way up to full participation."

"Just how am I supposed to start sex slowly and work my way up to 'full participation,' Doc?" The old sardonic tone was back. "Sounds like working up to motherhood by getting a little more pregnant each time."

"I didn't mean it that way. You don't work up to full participation, you work up to unrestrained freedom."

"Now what does *that* mean?"

"After your first visit to my office—that is, in two to three weeks—I'll check you over, and if there are no problems, you can engage in what Shakespeare called 'silken dalliance.' "

"Silken dalliance! Hey, I like that. In my price range it would be nylon."

"Anyway, you can have sex, but with a few minor restraints and safeguards. As you get over the shock of finding yourself still alive and well each time, your self-confidence will return, you'll shed some restraints, and get used to the safeguards. In time you'll be back to your normal sex behavior, possibly even better."

"What are the restraints and safeguards?"

"The first safeguard is getting rid of overweight. You're on your way to doing that."

"Yeah. Less weight on the lady, right?"

"No. Matter of fact, there's going to be *no* weight on your lady for a while. No, the extra weight is an extra burden on your heart. The less weight you carry, the less your heart has to work, the more energy for—"

". . . That silken dalliance. For that I'll stay thin."

"Safeguard number two—your physical condition."

"We covered that. I'm bringing my weight down."

"I'm talking about muscle conditioning. That's another reason I want to get you started on an exercise program. It will not only strengthen your heart, your circulation, your lung power and muscles, it's also good for your sex life."

"I knew I was playing tennis all these years for a reason," Frank grinned.

"Kidding aside, it *has* helped. If you had been sedentary and sluggish before your heart attack. I wouldn't have encouraged sex for you until you had pulled yourself into physical shape, no matter how long it took."

"How long *is* it going to take?"

I looked at him, surprised. "I just told you. It can be right after your first checkup in the office in two or three weeks."

"Oh, yeah. Great," he said, not looking like it would be great at all.

"What's the matter? You know I'm not going to send you up for that first flight until I'm sure the engine's in working order."

"Oh, sure."

"Frank, do you enjoy sex with your wife?"

He blinked. "What? Of course. I've enjoyed it for twenty years."

"And you like her."

"Like my wife? Hell, I love her."

"Very good."

He looked at me oddly. "That's a funny question, Doc—'do I like my wife.' "

"You'd be surprised how many men secretly dislike their wives and still enjoy sex with them. In fact, some psychiatrists say that part of the enjoyment these men have is because of their hostility."

"It takes all kinds, doesn't it? But there won't be any hostility with Sheila. Maybe there won't be anything at all."

"What does that mean?"

"Come on, Harold. After twenty years it gets a little tame with one's wife, wouldn't you say?"

"Not necessarily. I've got a woman patient who still has to lock her husband out of the bathroom when she takes a bath or he'll make a pass at her. She's seventy-two and he's seventy-five."

"Maybe that's the secret. Locking your husband out of the bathroom. Anyway, with mě it's, ah . . . ."

"Familiar?"

"Right!"

"Terrific." He looked to see if I was being sarcastic. "Frank, we've been talking about your return to sex as though you were a prize fighter returning to the ring. But that's only part of the story. Sex is an emotional as well as physical act, so you've got to have psychological safeguards, too. One should select the right partner when starting sexual activities after a heart attack."

"She's got to be able to turn him on, right?" He sounded almost pleading.

"Important, but the least important."

"The least important?" He looked shocked. "What the hell's the most important?"

"Familiarity. The best possible mate for a sexual comeback after a heart attack is someone with whom the patient has had long, satisfactory sex relations."

"You mean like my wife?"

"Well, is she the one with whom you've had the longest, most satisfactory sex relations?" I said, deadpan.

"That's a hell of a question to ask a happily married man."

"I ask pretty much the same question of divorced men, bachelors, widowers, divorcees, spinsters, widows, happy or unhappy."

Frank sighed. "Yeah, sure, it's Sheila. But by now it's it's, ah . . ."

"Twenty years."

"Yeah, you know what I mean."

"Frank, when you do play tennis again are you going to start with a tournament singles opposite the club professional?"

He stared at me. "Tournament singles? Harold, I'm not crazy."

"O.K. Well, getting back into sex after a heart attack is taxing enough for a married man without the added tension of starting with an illicit relationship."

He tried a feeble joke. "Doc, are you insinuating I'm planning to go to bed with a pro?"

"No pros, Frank, no mistresses and no office romances."

"Hey, you are beginning to sound like my rabbi."

"Do I? Well, get a load of this. The best sex advice for married heart patient to follow is the Seventh Commandment."

"Which one is that?"

" 'Thou shalt not commit adultery.' Medically, it's damn good advice."

Frank was quiet a moment. Then he said, "Take it slow with someone you know."

"Hey, that's good, Frank. It would make a great slogan if they ever formed a post-cardiac Masters and Johnson sex life institute. 'Take it slow with someone you know.' "

"And I could do the drawings to go with it," Frank grinned.

"Absolutely. Well, that finishes my sex talk for today."

"Don't go yet, Doc."

"You've got a visitor waiting."

"That's what I want to talk to you about." He paused. "She isn't just here because she's nice enough to visit her boss in the hospital. She's here because I phoned her and asked her to visit."

"Oh, I see," I said, straight-faced.

"I was going to try and fix up a date with her at a motel after I'm out of the hospital. You know. Like I told you, I've been thinking of sex a lot these past days and I've been scared. You might say I was scared about being scared." He was letting it all out in a tumble of words. "I figure I climb into bed, it's the first time after my heart attack and suppose I'm so scared by that—there I am with my wife and I can't get it up. So I figure it's a safer bet to kick off my return to sex by starting with a girl who is so sexy she could turn on anybody."

"You're afraid of being impotent that first time."

He didn't look at me as he nodded. "Doc, I'm more scared of flunking out in the kip than I am of having a heart attack there."

"Frank, there's a lot more chance of the first happening than the second."

He looked alarmed. "I may be impotent?"

"Impotent is an awfully strong word. Let's put it this way: you go to have sex for the first time after a heart attack, sure, you're going to have a fear of having a heart attack during intercourse. That fear can happen to any male cardiac. It's easier for the woman, since she can just lie there until she's caught up in it. I smiled. "Sort of seduced during the sex act."

Frank didn't smile.

"But, for obvious reasons, it's not that easy for a man."

"Obvious is right," Frank said. "It shows."

"Right. If a man is too worried, he won't have an erection. Usually he gets over the fear in a minute. But sometimes it takes a couple of tries before he's relaxed enough to perform satisfactorily. And, Frank, it can happen just as readily with a sex pot as with a wife."

"It can?"

"That impotence comes out of your fear, not out of your response to your partner."

"I hadn't thought of that."

"O.K., suppose you fail in front of your wife that first time. How much will that bother you? You've been married a long time, you've had all those years together, she's been with you through all your ups and downs—"

"That's for sure," Frank couldn't resist.

"... But suppose you flunk out with your model friend?"

He looked horrified. "My God, that's what happened with the first girl I ever had, or tried to have. I was sixteen. It set me back years."

"Familiarity has its points, wouldn't you say?"

"No question. Got any other pointers?"

"Yes, but it can keep." I nodded toward the door. "You've got someone waiting."

"Don't worry. She's on time and a half."

"O.K. The principle to keep in mind is that you're going to make everything as easy on your heart as possible. So before that first encounter, make sure you're well rested. In fact, it might be a good idea to arrange the initial rendezvous for late at night or the morning after a good night's sleep."

"Well, all right," Frank said slowly. "I generally feel a lot more like it in the evening."

"That's all right. Just make sure it's at least two to three hours after your last meal. We won't want your heart working on digesting your last meal and your first inter- course at the same time."

"God forbid," he said piously.

"And in those three hours in between do a lot of resting."

"What about having a couple of drinks?"

"You can have a drink at the meal or some wine."

"I'm talking about a couple of shots before we go into action. It would help, you know."

"Well, if you drink just enough to relax you, fine. It might smooth out your tension to the point where you can achieve an erection easily. But you've got to know how much just enough is. You keep drinking past that point, and—how did Shakespeare put it? 'It increaseth the desire but taketh away the performance.' Too much alcohol can make it difficult to achieve an erection and you can exhaust yourself with foreplay. Or you can start feeling overconfi- dent of your sexual prowess—"

"Cocksure," Frank interjected, straightfaced.

". . . You get high, you initiate things in bed you have no business trying as yet . . ."

"O.K., how about just a glass of wine?"

"And one for your wife. You don't stop being a gentle- man just because you're taking her to bed."

"Gentleman, hell! I'm going to put her in charge of the bottle."

"Very smart. Now, some small points. Make sure the temperature of the room is comfortable. If it's too hot or too cold, the heart has to work harder to keep the body temperature normal."

"Doc," Frank said unhappily, "you keep talking about

not letting the heart work too hard. Suppose the heart *is* working too hard. How will I know?"

"You may get chest pains or unusual shortness of breath."

"What should I do then?"

"What would you do if you were taking a brisk walk and you felt chest pains, or if you were in the middle of your exercises or in the middle of an argument and that happened? You would quit whatever you're doing and rest."

"You mean stop sex then and there? No orgasm?"

"Right. Chest pains take precedence over pleasure. Of course, the chest pains may have nothing to do with your heart. It may not be angina. It may be some kind of a muscular reaction. I'd be able to tell you that the next time you were in my office."

Frank's expression was unhappy. "I'm liable to get angina pains while I'm—"

"Frank, you should always keep a few nitroglycerin tablets near you, like on the night table next to your bed. All you have to feel is the first twinge of anything and you reach over for one of those tablets and pop it under your tongue."

"What'll it do?"

"If it's angina, in a matter of seconds, no chest pains."

"Yeah, but aren't those chest pains a warning system? I mean, the pill cuts out the chest pains so you keep going when you shouldn't?"

"Like taking out a road sign that says 'Bridge Out Ahead' so you keep driving and go crash? It's nothing like that. Angina pains come because a section of the heart temporarily doesn't get enough blood. The nitroglycerin dilates the narrowed coronary vessels so that the blood can get through easily. In other words, the tablet doesn't just cut out the pain of the condition. It actually *relieves* the condition causing the pain. So, have no fear about putting a nitroglycerin tablet under your tongue in the middle of lovemaking. I've got some information on that and other stuff in a guide I've prepared."

"You got one on you?"

". . . Which I just happen to have on me." I smiled as I handed him one.

He skimmed it rapidly. "About positions. The woman runs the show, huh?"

"In your case, yes. For a while."

"What do you mean—in my case?"

"Well, you're a man. For a while, you'll have to be the one catered to. Lie on your back, all that sort of thing. A woman recovering from a coronary, of course, usually doesn't have to change her ways."

"I see that."

"Frank, it's not a question of who runs the show. I told you the first principle of your comeback is making things as easy for your heart as possible. Especially in the initial phases."

Frank looked off pensively into the distance. "There's a kid joke I remember about the bride describing sex to a virgin friend. 'I lie there like a princess and he's up there working himself into a lather.' Now I'm the one who's going to be lying there like a princess." He didn't sound happy.

"Frank, when you have a chance to think it through, you'll understand just how little labels mean in a situation like this. What's important is just being comfortable as you go through this initial period of adjustment. That's why it makes much more sense to start your sexual activities with someone who is familiar to you, whom you like a lot and who doesn't judge you or provoke guilt. See, at this juncture, your wife has many roles to play in your life. Your coronary may do a lot to strengthen your relationship."

"Jesus, Doc, you're beginning to make it sound like no marriage ought to be without a coronary."

"No, but if you do have one, you might as well let it work for you, build a better second life, to help you both become better, more understanding companions."

Frank shrugged. "Maybe you've got something."

I stood up. "See you tomorrow."

"Right. On your way out, would you tell Melanie she can come in now."

"All right."

"And, Doc, leave the door open all the way, huh? The shorter the visit, the better. Then back to the shop for her. After all, she's on time and a half."

13. It Takes Two

"I wish I were lying there instead of Frank," Sheila Justin had said to me a week after her stricken husband had entered the hospital. At the time she said this, he was still in the Coronary Care Unit. At my request, she had stopped by my office on her way to her daily vigil at the hospital—ten minutes of seeing Frank as he lay wired to various machines, then fifty minutes of waiting in the lounge or coffee shop, until the next ten-minute visit. I was touched by what appeared to be a statement of self-sacrificing sentiment until she added, "God, could I use the rest!"

Then it all came pouring out. The eight-year-old had started bed-wetting. Margot, thirteen, had had her first asthma attack since kindergarten. Alex was "going around pale as a ghost, poor darling."

"If you knew how little sleep I've had since his attack. You know there are times I think Frank did this to me deliberately and I hate him for it." She looked at me with great, guilty eyes. "I'm awful, aren't I?"

She was wearing a cotton dress that needed pressing and there were dark rings under her eyes, which she had half-heartedly tried to conceal with make-up.

I shrugged. "You're just being normal."

"Normal!" She stared at me. "While my husband's in the hospital I'm carrying on about myself—that's normal?"

"Well, who else would carry on for you? There's a great line in *Death of a Salesman*. The one the wife says about her harassed husband: 'Attention must be paid to this man.' But harassed women need attention and sympathy, too, even if sometimes they have to get it from themselves."

"I don't know why I need any sympathy. I'm not facing this alone. After all, I have my family helping me." She sighed.

I decided it was time to give her the news I had invited her to my office to hear.

"This afternoon Frank is going to be transferred from CCU to a regular hospital room."

She brightened. "That means he's really getting better, doesn't it?"

"Indeed he is. It means the chances of complications have been reduced to the point where he doesn't have to be under constant observation."

She gave a great sigh of relief. "Won't he be thrilled!"

"Maybe, but I wouldn't count on it. Not for a day or two at least."

She looked at me, incredulous. "But every time I see him he takes half our ten minutes complaining about being plugged into all those wires."

"He complains to me, too. But lying there, taped to all those tubes, with those machines monitoring the heart around the clock, gives most heart patients a great sense of being protected. Moving out of that coronary room can be like moving out of a cradle for an infant."

"Do you mean he'll be unhappy about it?"

"You ask him, he'll probably tell you it's just fine. But if I were you I'd play it cool. Don't make a big fuss about the move. If he's secretly apprehensive about it, and you jump for joy, it might irritate him. Just tell him how well he's doing, how well he's looking . . ."

"He *is* doing well, isn't he?"

"Absolutely great. We wouldn't be moving him out of CCU if he weren't. His heart's mending, the EKG is improving—"

"How soon will he be home?" she blurted out. Then she blushed. "I just keep asking that same question, don't I?"

"It's perfectly natural, Sheila."

"Well, I'm ashamed. I mean if I were all alone I could understand. But God knows everyone's rallied around. My sister's at my house every day, my mother's moved in to help with the children. I don't know what I'd do without them." She fidgeted with her purse. "Though I wish my mother wasn't always walking around with such a long face. You can imagine what that does to the children."

"Why don't you say something to her about it?"

"Oh, Mother is sensitive, and it isn't as though she actually *says* anything in front of the kids. It's that frightened look she has and the way she keeps sighing like it's the end of the world."

"Maybe your sister could get it across to her."

"My . . . sister." Sheila spaced the words out coldly. "You know what she said to me this morning? 'Sheila, darling, whatever you do, don't feel guilty about Frank's heart attack.' Can you imagine!"

"There's no reason you should."

"But until she said it to me, I hadn't even thought about it. Now I can't get it out of my mind. Am I guilty?"

"Absolutely not." I said firmly. "People have coronaries because of a combination of things—what they eat and drink, how they work and play, their weight, their exercise, their temperament, their egos, their anxieties, their ambitions, their hates, their heredity. The importance of each factor in the combination varies from person to person. In essence what's crucial to the heart is not so much what happens to the heart's owner but how the owner reacts. So stop feeling guilty. You're not the cause of Frank's coronary, but once Frank has returned to his new life, a lot of the responsibility for not letting it happen again will rest with you."

"Oh, I'm ready for that," she glowed. "I feel so much better. Lisa's crack upset me so."

"She probably meant well."

"Oh, she always means well. Her favorite line is 'I'm doing the best I know how.' She was great the first two days, but now I'm getting the feeling she's beginning to enjoy running our lives. She likes to take over."

"Given the chance, a lot of people do."

"Not like Lisa. Even when we were kids she was bossy." She laughed apologetically. "I guess I shouldn't be telling you all this, Doctor."

"Better to tell me now than Frank later."

"Oh, I'm always cheerful with Frank. I tell him everything's just fine. But, you know something, he can always see through me. I wonder why."

I searched for a diplomatic way to answer her question. "Has it occurred to you that what Frank sees is more convincing than what you tell him?"

"What do you mean?"

"Well," I cleared my throat. "Is it possible that the reason you don't sort of, ah . . ."—I groped and came up with a lame phrase—"fix yourself up before you go see Frank is because you're trying to convey to him what a tough time you're having at home all by yourself?"

She looked shocked, then pulled a compact from her bag and studied her face. "My God, what a rotten job I did under my eyes." She tried to tuck in some tendrils of hair. "Maybe you're right. Maybe I am trying to show him how rough it is at home. But why would I do that?"

"Why do you think?"

She stared at the mirror, making ineffectual primping gestures, then stopped. "I hate to admit this, but I wouldn't be surprised if I was trying to make him feel guilty. Sick as he is." She gave me a wry look. "Don't tell me that's normal too, Doctor."

"I'll tell you what's normal, Sheila. Once there's been a coronary in a marriage, it's never the same marriage again. It can't be. There's a threat and a fright that shifts things. But it's the great opportunity of the marriage. If you accept the challenge, you learn to cope and to handle and to give. You'll grow and so will your marriage."

Sheila studied herself again. "I'm pretty sure they'll squeeze me in at the beauty shop," she said, more to the mirror than me. "Then I'll go home and change"—she smiled at me and stood up—"and 'fix myself up.' If you see Frank, tell him I'll be a little late. After all, with him just getting out of Coronary Care, I'm dressing up for his coming-out party."

"Maybe it's *your* coming-out party too."

The next time I saw her in my office more than a week later, it was at her request. I could hardly recognize the weary, slightly bedraggled Sheila of the previous Monday. It was not only the smartness of her outfit and the make-up, it was her manner, which was now easy and confident. She carried some library books.

"You look great, Sheila. Well rested."

"I'm so busy all day I sleep well at night out of sheer exhaustion."

"How are things going?"

"Fine." There was no brave, sympathy-seeking smile this time. "I finally did tell my mother about her gloomy look and how it was affecting the children. Now she's Mary Sunshine. That gets a little wearing at times, but it's a lot better than the gloom."

"What about the kids?"

"Coming along beautifully. I've organized them into work squads for every chore in the house from gardening to cooking. Alex is in charge. They're all doing their bit for Dad, I tell them, and you know something? It's working."

"That's probably the best thing you could do for them."

"And for me. It gave me a graceful reason to cut down on Lisa's visits. I told her how important it was for the kids to be on their own with a minimum of adult supervision. Giving children a sense of unsupervised responsibility is a good idea, don't you think?"

"Yes."

"I'm glad you feel that way, because I told Lisa it was your idea. If it came from me, she might not have taken it." Then she deftly changed the subject. "Doctor, one of the things I've come to see you about are these books on the heart I'm bringing to Frank."

"Nothing wrong with him reading heart books. Matter of fact—"

"That's not what's bothering me. You see, the first few days after Frank got out of Coronary Care, his accountant was getting all these books out of the library for him. Then suddenly he switched the job to me. It's not as though his accountant was overworked."

"Are you?"

"Oh, I can fit it in, but that's not the point. Frank keeps piling little jobs on me. Like he wants freshly laundered pajamas every other day. I don't mind it, I like it; but he's gotten so critical about everything—like if the pajamas aren't pressed or if I don't get him the book just when he wants it. It's nine days since he's been out of Coronary Care. Shouldn't he be over being cranky about leaving there by now?"

"Oh, he was over that last week. Now he's unhappy about just being in the hospital. He's taking it out on you."

"But not on anyone else."

"Of course not. You're his wife. He loves you."

She shot me a quick look to see if I was joking. However, I wasn't.

"He certainly has a funny way of showing it. When he was in Coronary Care, he was so worried I wouldn't be able to handle things without him. Now that I've got things under control, I thought he'd be tickled. Instead he's gotten so crabby and demanding.".

She pulled a small sealed jar from her handbag and displayed it. "Look what he's got me doing."

"What is it?"

"Fruit salad. One portion. They've got it on the hospital menu, but he insists I make some fresh every day and bring it to him. I offered to make him a big jar and the nurse could put it away in the refrigerator and give him some every day, but, no, he wants me to make it fresh."

"Has Frank ever done anything like this since you've known him?"

"You mean did he ever ask me to make him fruit salad every day?"

"Well, did he ever insist on you doing something special for him regularly?"

"Like what?"

"Like, let's say, give him a back rub, phone him at a certain time each day, anything like that?"

She started to shake her head, then said hesitantly, "Well, when we first met and started dating, Frank was drafted and sent to Germany for a year. If he didn't get a letter from me every day at his post, he'd get really upset."

"Why?"

She shrugged. "It's easy to understand. He was young, he was lonely, so my letters meant something to him."

"What do you mean by 'something'?"

She looked impatient.

"They meant I loved him."

"You mean they reassured him that you loved him."

"Well, isn't that the same thing?"

"It's a little more, and in this case that little more is important. There's Frank lying on his back fretting about how his wife is going to manage things without him. After a heart attack a man may feel terribly insecure, useless. Well, when his wife suddenly starts handling things well and looking well in the bargain, one would think he would be relieved. Actually, now he feels twice as worthless, and he feels about as far away from you as when he was in Germany. He wants that fruit salad made by you for him every day to give him the same reassurance you gave him when he was in the service."

Sheila looked down at the fruit salad. "My letters to Germany," she said and began to cry.

At my request, Sheila came to my office again the following week. It was the day before Frank was to return home for his convalescence.

"Don't try to turn the house into a hospital with you as the nurse," I told her. "The last thing Frank wants is any more of that hospital atmosphere. Just be alert to his needs."

"And give him a lot of tender loving care," Sheila said.

"That'll help. Also, the medicines he has to take—keep at least an extra three-day supply separate as an emergency measure."

"Emergency?" She looked apprehensive.

"In case he runs out of something on a Sunday or a Friday night and your drugstore isn't open."

"That makes sense."

"As a routine precaution, get the phone number where you can get help fastest to your house. It's probably the fire department in your neighborhood."

"Yes, it is."

"O.K. Then post a list of emergency phone numbers near each phone in your house where they can be easily seen. First, the fire department rescue squad, then my phone number, then any other numbers you would call in case of an emergency. After all, you might not be home if one of the children or Frank had an emergency."

Sheila nodded, still tense.

"Sheila," I said, "do you carry fire insurance on your house?"

"Of course," she answered, surprised. "What has that got to do with—"

"Well, the chances of your needing it are slight, but you wouldn't think of not carrying it. And the chances of Frank needing any of these precautions are even slighter, but it's still insurance."

She nodded and smiled. "I understand."

"Now, the first week or so Frank may spend much of his time in bed. I suggest you have some kind of communication system from the bedroom. Do you have a telephone intercom or a loud dinner bell?"

"Is that in order to save his voice?"

"I doubt if Frank will feel much like yelling the first day or two. Also, conceivably a situation could arise where he feels too weak to yell."

Sheila looked alarmed again. "Sheila, I'm not expecting anything like that, but after a coronary I take the Boy Scout motto as my creed—'Be prepared.' Speaking of Boy Scouts, I'd take a class in life saving and heart resuscitation, if I were you." Her eyebrows started to go up again. "Sheila, I told you I'm not expecting anything, but these days it's an easy skill to acquire in a matter of a few hours at your convenience. You can find out where classes are being held through the Red Cross or the American Heart Association or the Y or the fire department. It might come in handy some day at the beach or at a swimming pool."

"Can my son take the course?"

"Alex? Certainly. And so can your daughter. They should know what to do if they're faced with an emergency like a drowning or a heart attack. It's a handy skill these days."

"Doctor, somebody told me I ought to have a portable oxygen inhalator in the house, just in case."

I shrugged. "If it gives you a feeling of reassurance, get one. Frank certainly doesn't need oxygen. But I'll give you a little tip about oxygen that most people don't know."

"What?"

"Great for hangovers," I whispered.

It was a pleasure to watch her laugh.

Next day, eighteen days after I had rushed him into the hospital with the first symptoms of a myocardial infarction, Frank was ready to go home. On his final morning I told him most of the jeopardy was behind him, his heart was healing well, and chances of a relapse were extremely slim. He should remember FDR's famous line that the only thing to fear was fear itself. Finally, I said, he would undoubtedly be able to return to work, at least part-time, within a month.

"A *month!*" he exclaimed. "Didn't you say three weeks?"

"I said within a month."

"And how soon will I be playing tennis?"

"Within six months."

"How about three months?"

"Come on, Frank, you're not negotiating with a buyer. Still if you keep improving at this rate anything is possible."

His wife drove him home.

Two weeks later she brought him to the office for his first post-hospital checkup. He came out of the examination room and sat down carefully in one of the two upholstered chairs that faced my desk. Sheila stood behind him. I told him his heart appeared to be healing at an excellent rate. "You must be following all my directions."

"To the letter, Doctor. Diet, exercise, recreation, everything. He squeezed Sheila's fingers which were on his shoulder. "She checks me with whips in both hands."

Sheila beamed. I told Frank to start increasing his activities and said that after another week he could go to his office for a few hours each day. He was to go in the late morning after having rested at least one hour after breakfast, spend no more than two hours at work, and then to come home for lunch and stay home the rest of the day.

"Hey, that's great, Doc!" he said.

It was only after they had left, with Sheila solicitously opening and closing doors, that I realized that this was the first time I could remember in the last five weeks that Frank hadn't brought up the subject of tennis. He also hadn't once challenged me or made a ribbing remark. And he had stopped calling me by my first name. I was now "Doctor" or "Doc."

The next checkup came two weeks later. Again Sheila drove him in, and stood behind him as he sat in the office. I asked him how his first week at work had gone.

"I haven't gone back yet," he said. "Sheila and I felt maybe we ought to get this next checkup under our belt before I start work." She nodded approvingly.

"Not a bad idea," I said cautiously. Frank wasn't talking like Frank when he said "*we* ought to" and "under *our* belt." His personality had sobered. He was interested in all the details of his case. What was his blood pressure and how did it compare with that of two weeks ago? What was his cholesterol count? His pulse? He asked educated questions about his EKG.

"I didn't realize what a close shave I had," he said, as though apologizing for his new attitude.

"I've seen considerably closer that have made excellent recoveries," I told him. "We have patients who have been longshoremen, truck drivers, workers in heavy industry. Many of them have been able to return to full-time heavy labor after they've recovered from the myocardial infarction. I see no reason why you should not be able to do anything and everything you've ever done in the past after you've fully recovered."

Frank waited politely until I'd finished. "Sheila brought

me some insurance statistics," he said. "Do you know that ten years after a coronary, a large percentage of coronary cases are dead?"

"I wouldn't worry about it, Frank. Most of those deaths occur in patients in their late sixties, seventies, and even eighties. Who knows how many would have lived ten years more, even if they hadn't had coronaries?"

Sheila patted Frank's shoulder. "It's just a matter of being careful, darling. Isn't that right, Doctor?"

"Not too careful," I cautioned. "Otherwise you can turn into a hypochondriac, a cardiac cripple, Frank. By stopping smoking, bringing your weight down, reducing the tension in your life, and coming in here periodically for a checkup, you make your chances of a recurrent heart attack go way down. You know, from 1940 on, coronary deaths for men were rising spectacularly. Then we started to get people to lose weight, stop smoking, reduce tensions in their life and control high blood pressure. Result: since 1968 there's been a dramatic drop in coronary deaths for men between the ages of thirty-five to sixty-four." I smiled at Sheila. "Physicians must be doing something right, wouldn't you say?"

Looking tenderly at Frank she nodded absently.

The next scheduled checkup was six weeks after Frank had been released from the hospital. Sheila was still his chauffer-companion. I asked him if he had returned to work. He nodded. "Yep. I go in two or three days a week like you told me."

I didn't bother telling him that he was a good three weeks behind schedule. "Full days?"

"No, half days. There's no sense rushing it, is there?"

While he was having his EKG and chest x-ray, I had a few minutes alone with Sheila in my office.

"Frank seems to have changed quite a bit, wouldn't you say?"

"Oh, yes. And it wasn't easy getting him to, Doctor. You remember how do-it-yourself he was."

"Indeed."

"The first day I brought him breakfast in bed, he kicked up such a fuss. I must have spent half an hour getting through to him that it was important to help his heart. It's taken a lot of doing, but you see how he's changed," she said proudly.

"Do you like him better this way?"

"Oh, yes." She added softly, "He's more mine."

"That's a lovely way of putting it, Sheila. Like a mother talking about her children. The younger the child is, the more it belongs to her."

That got through. She looked at me askance. "Oh, I didn't mean anything like Frank being a child."

"What did you mean?"

"I meant we're a lot closer than we were."

"Well, a mother is a lot closer to the infant in her arms than she is, let's say, to the child who's already going to school."

"Are you saying that I'm babying Frank?"

"What do *you* think?"

"Doctor, Frank is recovering from a heart attack!"

"Physically, he's almost recovered. Psychologically, he's had a relapse."

"A relapse?"

"Even when he was in Coronary Care, more than two months ago, his major interest was how long before he would be out and ready to pick up his life where he had left off. Seven weeks out of the hospital and he's still dropping in to his business place only two or three times a week."

"Maybe he isn't as interested in his business as he was before his attack," Sheila said. "When he was in the hospital, didn't you tell him to find things to enjoy rather than to compete in?"

"Yes. It's one of the good things someone can get out of an ordeal like a heart attack. Get a better idea of what life is all about and change their way of living accordingly. Well, what's Frank's lifestyle now? What does he do with himself all day?"

"Well, he gets up in the morning, about nine . . ."

"Does he see the children?"

"No, they're already in school, but he does see them when they get home."

"Anyway, you get him up, take his pulse and temperature, record them on a chart you've rigged up next to the bed."

"Did Frank tell you?"

"Yes. You bought him a sphygmomanometer so he could take his blood pressure whenever he wants to. You do all the driving, even though I told him to start driving a week ago. You serve him breakfast in bed—not only in the morning but all day long. Emotionally, he doesn't *want* to get out of bed."

"Doctor, I do the best I know how."

"Wasn't that what your sister said to you when she was coming over to your house to help? 'I'm doing the best I know how.' Didn't you tell me she's the sort of person who likes to take over? And didn't I tell you a lot of people do, *given the chance?*"

Sheila fidgeted unhappily. "It's a lot different with Frank and me than it was with my sister and me. I resented Lisa, but Frank doesn't resent me. In fact, he's grateful."

"Frank had a heart attack. Unless you've had one, it's hard to conceive the apprehension that goes on inside the heart victim, no matter how much bravado they show the world."

"I would think a person who has any serious illness has apprehension."

"But no other part of the body has the emotional meaning of the heart. I mean, we know eyes are for seeing, ears are for hearing, but a heart isn't just for pumping blood. Look at how it comes out in the language. A heart swells with pride, fills with gratitude, with longing, with dread, with rage. A heart softens, hardens. Have a heart. Don't break my heart. What I'm saying, Sheila, is that when a man has a heart attack, his dependence on his spouse drastically increases. In a way, he's at her mercy and sometimes it takes a lot of self-control for the wife not to take advantage of it."

"Are you telling me that I'm taking advantage of Frank?"

"I'm speaking of wives in general. Sometimes, a husband's heart attack gives a wife the chance to play the martyr. As she's taking care of him, she lets him know how hard everything is on her. She loads him with enough guilt to sink an aircraft carrier. Then there are women who hate the role of nurse and they don't bother hiding it and they give their convalescing husband a great sense of being a burden."

"I don't hate the role of nurse, not when it comes to my family. In fact, I enjoy it."

"Maybe a little too much. It's possible to baby a strong man who feels dependent on you to the point where he starts feeling helpless about everything. Eventually, he'll resent it. It may be an enjoyable relationship but it's a far lesser one than that of man and wife."

"You mean it's my fault?"

Her stricken look reminded me of her expression the day

she had asked me if she were guilty of her husband's heart attack. I couldn't help smiling.

"Sheila, I wish you know how many dozens of wives sit in that same chair and ask me that same question every year. And how many husbands.

"Husbands?"

"Wives get heart attacks too."

"Of course." She gave a mirthless laugh. "I'd forgotten."

"That's understandable. In your and Frank's age bracket, about four times as many men have heart attacks as women. The husbands of cardiacs react pretty much the same as you wives. In fact, a lot of times, it's even easier for the man to be overprotective, overhelpful. When I point out to them that they're in danger of turning their wives into cardiac cripples, they ask the same thing, 'You mean, it's my fault?' "

"Well, *is* it my fault?"

One couldn't say Sheila wasn't singleminded.

"No, it isn't your fault. It takes two to tango. You offered Frank the excuse to stay comfortable as an invalid. He took it. Frank's a big boy. He could have turned it down."

She sighed. "You know, a lot of times, it's hard to figure out what to do."

"That's for sure. In convalescence, the best rule is to take the scaffolding away slowly, cautiously, and consistently. You know, mother-child situations don't only happen to wives of cardiacs. They happen to doctors, too." She looked at me surprised. "A lot of patients stay dependent on their doctor long after they should. They keep phoning in about every insignificant cold or scratch or ache. I give them the specific reassurance they have called me about, but, tacitly, I try to educate them regarding the exact importance or unimportance of their problem so they can have a proper perspective on the symptom the next time it occurs. In time, it dawns on most of them that they are not using me as a doctor but as a crutch. They realize they are now well enough to begin using their own judgment in specific familiar problems or situations. They aren't just dependent patients any more, they're partners, and it no longer seems right to whimper every time they scrape their knee. Better they should let out an oath and get on with life."

Later, I gave Frank his clean bill of health, "You're doing fine, Frank."

He turned to his wife. "I owe it all to this here broad."

"Thanks, honey. Let's go." She smiled and held out the car keys to him. "You drive."

14. The Good Jackals

"But you *must* remember him," I said to the croupier. "I left him playing here only seven or eight minutes ago!"

The Las Vegas stickman shook his head. I couldn't believe it.

"He was rolling dice for at least an hour!"

"People roll dice here all day, all night." His eyes watched the green baize on which cubes richocheted and tumbled. "I don't look at them. I look at the dice."

"Listen, he wouldn't have moved from here. We were doing a medical test. I'm a doctor."

The croupier's eyes flicked over me for just an instant, then back to the crap table.

"I didn't see him, mister." That 'mister' conveyed just how much stock he took in my story about being a doctor. "Maybe he's in the men's room."

"No, that's where I was. Look, he wouldn't have gone away without letting me know. He was my patient."

It was true he was my patient, and had been for the last twenty-two hours. We had met at a party in Beverly Hills the previous evening, and in the course of a twenty-minute conversation he had managed to play havoc with my usually well-regulated existence.

Christopher Blake was a stock speculator, or more correctly, since he had attained a seat on the New York State Exchange, a Wall Street financier. During a typical day, he bought and sold in large lots often on the basis of only a fractional anticipated change in the stock value. Frequently, the buy or sell order had to be timed so close to the fluctuations of the price on the big board that a difference of seconds in putting the order through could determine the profitability of the transaction.

Blake was thus under great tension in his work. During one of his high-stake maneuvers, amid the jangling of phones and the confusion of voices as his aides transmitted his orders, Blake would often find himself soaked with perspiration. And recently he had begun to find something more worrisome.

"When there's a crunch on," he said at the party, "I get these palpitations in my chest. Sometimes there's kind of a pressing or pinching pain, but it's so fleeting I can't even tell exactly where it is. Then when the tension is off, the palpitations go away and so does the pressing and the pinching. It bothers me."

"If it bothers you," I said politely, "you ought to go see your doctor when you get home. Lovely party, isn't it?"

I don't mind giving advice, but I avoid in-depth medical evaluations at social gatherings. A cocktail party diagnosis is at best a poor substitute for an office consultation and at worst a dangerous one. But either Blake didn't get my hint or he was displaying the same aggressiveness that had built him his financial empire.

"I've been gone over by three cardiologists in New York," he went on. "They've given me cardiograms and chest x-rays. They even put me on a treadmill, but they can't find anything wrong."

"Then what are you worrying about?"

"A lot of people say that to me, but you've got to remember that those three doctors checked me out in *their* offices, not mine. I wasn't under any pressure when I was in their places, so my electrocardiograms showed my heart was O.K., even when they exercised me." He sighed wearily. Tall and powerfully built, he looked more like an athletic coach than a tycoon. The air of weariness sat oddly on him.

"You know, a lot of times I feel maybe I'm like one of those old-time ship boilers. O.K. for ordinary steam, but if I ever get pushed up past a certain temperature—wham! I'll blow apart."

Blake was no fool. He realized the EKG's the doctors had taken represented less than one minute of his heartbeats, out of 1440 minutes in a day—only fifty or sixty heartbeats out of as many as 144,000 normal heartbeats daily. Even the stress test was a sampling of only ten or fifteen minutes. Though taken in carefully controlled fashion, the measurement was obviously limited, being recorded under the relatively artificial conditions of a doctor's office.

"You want to have your heart examined while you're under everyday office pressures, right?"

He nodded. "Right, Harold." He had put us on a first-name basis as soon as I displayed interest in his problem.

"But how could I have a doctor check me over while I'm working in my office, with everything going crazy like it usually does?"

I shrugged. "Easy. It was licked by the space program."

"What was?"

"Your problem. NASA had to find out how an astronaut's heart would stand up under the strain of a rocket launch and work in space *before* he went on the flight, so it's not too unlike your problem."

"Well, what did they do?"

"A bright bioengineer, Jeff Holter, developed a gadget called a Holter monitor. It's a tape recorder to record the heart action continuously over a period of many hours. NASA used it to monitor the astronauts' hearts during simulated space flights. By now, these recorders have been miniaturized to the point where they're the size of a hand-held cassette recorder, and they can record the electrocardiogram for up to twenty-four hours. An analyst with a specially designed computerized scanner then scans the tapes, checking each heartbeat for abnormal rhythms, skipped beats, or evidence of heart strain. The patient also keeps a diary synchronized to the tape, so whether you're eating, working, or sleeping, or if you have any symptoms, we can tell exactly what your heart was doing during those times."

"Where can I get one of them?"

"Many large hospitals have them, and most cardiologists have access to them. When you get back to New York, ask your doctor—"

"I don't have a regular doctor, and anyway I'm not going back to New York for another week."

I shrugged. After all, he was not my patient. I felt the same kind of relief a waiter must experience in noting that a difficult diner is at some other waiter's table. Blake must have sensed my reaction. His attitude became apologetic.

"I know I sound awfully impatient, but if you knew how much this thing bothers me." He heaved a great sigh and wagged his head. "Just one complete night's sleep without waking up and staring at the ceiling. Is that asking too much, Harold?"

Pathos was his strong suit, no question. I couldn't help admiring the skillful way he used it. One felt moved and conned at the same time.

"Look, Mr. Blake—"

"Christopher," he corrected me.

"Look, Christopher—"

"My friends call me Chris."

"Look, Christopher, what would be the point of getting you a recorder when you have to go back to New York to use it since that's where you get the pains and palpitations? You can rent one in New York."

"Why do I have to go back to New York to use it? Can't we simulate that situation out here?" I stared at him. "After all," he went on glibly, "NASA simulated a rocket launch to test the astronauts wearing that gadget. Why can't we simulate the situation that brings on my palpitations?"

I don't know which bothered me more—the impracticality of his thinking or the presumptuousness of his "Why can't *we* . . . ?"

"Let me tell you something, Mr. Blake . . ." I said tartly. After all, this man wasn't my patient, in fact he wasn't even sick, just irritating. Then, suddenly, it came to me, out of the blue, the solution. "Chris," I said, "how would you describe your business in just one word?"

He shrugged. "Speculating."

"How about 'gambling'?"

"Sure. Playing the market's just a high-class crap shoot."

"So there s your answer! You want to simulate the pressures of your New York office? Get one of those Holter monitors, tape it onto your chest, go to Las Vegas, and shoot craps."

If I was exhilarated at my ingenuity, Blake was estatic.

"Sensational! Harold, you're fantastic! How soon can I get one of those Holter monitors?"

I shrugged. "Could be as early as tomorrow morning if you find a cardiologist willing to take you on as a patient. It's very easy for him to arrange to rent a Holter from a laboratory."

"Wonderful! We could leave for Las Vegas by noon."

"Who's we?"

"You and me. You're my doctor."

"Hold on a minute . . ."

"Money is no object, you understand." It was hard to believe anyone still talked that way.

"Right you are, Chris," I said, sarcastically. "Money is no object. At least not to me. My patients are my object, and my responsibility is to them."

"Look, why don't you take me on as a patient, give me a complete heart checkup? I don't have a regular doctor, you know."

"All right," I said with a sigh. "I'll get you your Holter and before you leave for Las Vegas, I'll be happy to fit it on you. It's just about as difficult as putting on a hearing aid. The only thing you have to remember when you're wearing it is to keep a diary. Every time you feel a symptom, write a short description of it and your activity and jot down the time it happened. These recorders have built-in clocks, and the time is recorded on a record track on the tape. When the cassette is completed, return everything to me. I'll get the tape analyzed and we'll find out exactly what your heart is doing while you're rolling dice."

"But, Harold, suppose while I'm playing, the excitement makes the old boiler blow and I keel over?"

Pure Wallace Berry dialogue.

"What you'd need then, of course, would be someone who's an expert at heart resuscitation."

"That's exactly what I mean."

"Well, you can hire yourself a trained male nurse who'll go along with you through the casino. In fact, he can make the entries in your diary for you."

Blake's face grew mournful.

"It wouldn't be the same thing, Harold. I mean having your own cardiologist around gives a patient a great sense of security."

"That's what all cardiac patients tell their cardiologists. And that's why I'm quite exhausted. I've had not only my own practice, but I've also been covering for a colleague out of the country. Also I've been on call three weekends in a row. Tomorrow, as a matter of fact, is the first Saturday I'm free to relax. So . . ." I paused and heard myself say, ". . . Chris, I think I'll go with you."

The whole concept of testing heart stresses at the gambling tables was becoming more and more fascinating to me. And of course it would be only proper to see the experiment to its conclusion. Besides, maybe I could work in a little time around the pool.

Next morning I had Blake hooked up to a Holter recorder at my office before we drove out to the airport. The technician carefully taped the three electrodes to his chest and then checked out the very thin, inconspicuous wire that connected the electrodes to the tape recorder. After Blake put his shirt back on, he looked at the recorder strapped to his belt with the wire running from it inside his shirt. He wagged his head in wonder.

"You look at this marvelous little gadget and you realize it comes of the space race. I mean if we hadn't been out to beat the Russians to the moon, it might never have been invented."

"Maybe so, maybe not. Wars always seem to stimulate industrial development. One branch of science develops devices to kill people and five or six years later, after the war is over, doctors come in and start to use those devices to diagnose or treat people. In this respect, the space effort was like a war. Maybe we should call ourselves the good jackals. An interesting example is nitroglycerin, which is one of the two most valuable heart drugs we have available to us. It was discovered while Paris was under siege during the Franco-Prussian War. A physician noticed that the French barricade fighters when hauling explosives, which are practically pure nitroglycerin, flushed beet-red and complained that their hearts were pounding. The physician had discovered the cardiovascular effects of nitroglycerin."

On the way to the airport, I told him about several wartime inventions that had recently been converted to use in cardiology. The sonarscope, a form of undersea radar used in the detection of submarines, substituted sound waves for radio waves had been adapted for medical use as the echocardiogram. "We can now study the structure of the heart without resorting to traumatic procedures or exploratory surgery," I explained. "We just send sound waves from outside the chest wall into the heart and record the waves that bounce back to the surface. We may eventually even be able to detect fatty deposits or obstructions building up in coronary arteries with this sonar-type device. In the future, we may be able to actually study the blood flow in the coronary arteries without the need of putting a catheter through the arteries and then taking an x-ray. Someday, hopefully, we'll be able to have a warning system which will detect the threat of a coronary thrombosis before it occurs. It'll be like our present ability to detect a hurricane build-up with satellites in orbit. In the case of detecting a heart attack threat, though, we'll be able to do a lot more about avoiding it then we can do about avoiding a hurricane." I was warming up to my subject. "Do you know what a sidewinder missile is?"

"Sure," Blake surprised me. "It's an antiballistic missile developed after World War II. It senses the heat being emitted from an enemy missile's engine, then it automatically sets its navigational devices and flies into the missile to destroy it." He grinned. "I owned stock in a company that manufactured missile parts. Now, how the hell can you use an antiballistic missile in the heart?"

"We don't. We use a modification of the heat-sensing unit in its nose cone and we call it a thermograph. We're warm-blooded animals and the heat variations over the surface of our bodies fluctuates constantly depending on many factors and in many situations it can alert us problems in certain parts of the body."

"You mean like having a fever," Blake said.

"The only heat-sensing device you need for a fever is a thermometer which, by the way, was invented by Galileo. A thermograph on the other hand, is so sophisticated it can record as many as a half million temperature variations of an area of the body in as little as one-sixteenth of a second. In fact, we're now able to take a Polaroid picture of a person, using the heat emission from their body instead of light. We can take this photograph in pitch blackness, the way the high-flying U-2 planes can take pictures of enemy troops at night. Studying those thermograph photographs, we're learning to read the state of health of various areas of the body. For instance, we can detect breast cancer that is too small to show up on x-rays."

"What about the heart?"

"We're moving along. For instance, because of the anatomical distribution of the blood vessels, some people who have a high risk of getting a stroke, may have relative coolness over one or both eyes which is related to a decrease in blood flow to the brain. We can easily detect this coolness with a thermographic examination. A group of us recently completed a project in association with the Bioengineering Department of RAND—you know, the think tank in Santa Monica—on a program that will eventually be used to detect people who might develop a certain kind of stroke. This potential stroke-screening unit will use thermography and other simple tests. No knives, no needles, no risks, no discomforts, and the study can be repeated as often as needed with no ill effects."

"Say, that's cool."

"Or hot," I smiled. "Anyway, it's thermography and our aim is to eventually eliminate or alter cardiovascular problems by detecting them at earlier stages."

"Listen," Blake said earnestly, "if you ever want to form a company on any of this, I'll be happy to donate my services absolutely free of charge. Or if you need any backing."

"How about a donation to the cardiology department at a medical school? Christopher Blake, patient and philanthropist."

"Besides," he grinned, "I can deduct it from my income tax."

When we arrived in Las Vegas, Blake insisted we check into a hotel, although we planned to fly back that night.

"It's a good idea," I said. "Give you a place to rest between rounds."

"That's not why I do it," Blake said. "What I do is take out all the money I intend to play with and then put my wallet with the rest of my money in the hotel safe. I don't redeem it until I've checked out. That way I'm not tempted to exceed my gambling budget."

It seemed like an excellent idea, and certainly within the character of a disciplined Wall Street financier. I didn't know that this time it would lead to his undoing.

"Another rule I have," Blake said, "is play at a casino as far away from that safe as I can get."

Twenty minutes later we were in a casino at the other end of the Strip and Blake was busy at the crap table. He played carefully and well. As he had told me, he had a finely honed grasp of the law of probability, and he used it with sophisticated skill, winning more often than he lost. He played for comparatively small sums, rarely more than fifty dollars on a roll of the dice, but it wasn't the amount that counted with him. As he had said at the party, "Money is no object." For him winning was the object. And it showed. Even though he played in a methodical, careful way, apparently cool and collected, inside he was not. He would grin when he won, bite his lips when he lost. Perspiration rolled from his forehead.

I never got to the pool. Since I was holding the patient diary, I didn't play. After all, I was keeping in mind that this was a dynamic electrocardiography test on a patient.

After Blake had secured the dice and had been throwing some three minutes, he turned to me, wiping the beads of sweat from his forehead and whispered, "I'm getting those palpitations now."

I jotted it down. A half hour later, after seven straight passes, during which people crowded around to watch, he turned to me, putting his handkerchief under his wilted sport shirt collar, and said, "They won't stop."

"Mild?" I asked.

"Yeah." He threw the dice. Another pass. People gasped and applauded. He turned to me. "Not so mild."

He had let his original bet ride and he had a mound of chips that was worth close to a thousand dollars. The momentum and excitement had by now mounted to an almost unbearable level. Unfortunately for me another matter had simultaneously mounted to an even more pressing level and I reluctantly told Blake I would have to take a break to the nearest men's room. He scarcely nodded, he was so intent on his game.

It was when I returned that I found him gone. After my dialogue with the croupier, who claimed he had never noticed Blake, I went to the pit boss. He claimed to be equally ignorant of Blake's whereabouts. I was beginning to feel like a character in an Alfred Hitchcock movie. As I was about to leave to inquire elsewhere, the pit boss said, almost as a casual afterthought, "You might try the office."

At the casino office, when I inquired about my missing patient, I was ushered into an inner office. Blake sat in a chair, his jacket and shirt off, his Holter monitor still hanging from his belt, and the wires still taped to his chest. He was surrounded by three bulky men.

As I walked in, he jumped up with relief, "Harold! Will

you tell these guys about this?" He indicated his Holter. "They think it's some kind of device for controlling dice."

It took a few words of explanation and showing my credentials to set everything straight. There were apologies all around. "You've got to understand, Doctor," the largest of the trio explained, "it wasn't only the fact that he was wearing that box—the stickman spotted it—but when we got him into the office he didn't have any identification on him."

We left the office. "Go ahead, laugh," Blake said sheepishly. "I've got it coming."

"Oh, no," I said, trying to hold my laughter in. "Actually, I'm to blame, too. I should have warned you to keep it better hidden. The incident in Minneapolis slipped my mind."

"What incident in Minneapolis?"

"Well, this goes back to the time the Weatherman radicals blew up a couple of public buildings and everybody got real jumpy. This patient went into a bank wearing a Holter device. The teller kept him waiting, the bank guard kept him in conversation, and suddenly a couple of men in screened masks and flak vests grabbed him and shoved him into a steel van and headed for a bomb deactivation chamber. What happened was that he was wearing an open-collared shirt and some of the wires on his Holter device could be seen across his chest. The bank people and the police thought that he was a walking bomb. He kept telling them it was an electrocardiographic recorder but they didn't take any chances. It took that special bomb squad forty-five minutes to ease the Holter unit off him, and get it to stop working."

By the time I finished the story, we were both laughing.

We returned to Los Angeles that same Saturday night. The following Monday, the tape, the Holter recorder, and the diary I had kept for Blake were sent over to the analytical laboratory. I invited the high roller to come over to the laboratory to watch the scanning and analysis of his "day at Las Vegas" tape. When we got to the lab, the tape had been analyzed and evaluated.

"Nothing but good news, Chris," I told him. "Your palpitations are nothing more than a physiological response to the excitement of the moment. They're like the rapid heart action of an athlete in a contest during periods of extreme pressure, or even the response of a spectator watching it and being carried away by the excitement. The same reaction can be detected in people who are in a state of apprehension . . ." I grinned. ". . . like when I came back from the men's room and found you had disappeared."

I went back and forth between the diary notes and Blake's EKG tape chart.

"It's interesting to note that at the time we left my office to go to the airport, your heart rate was only beating about eighty-six times per minute. When we arrived in Las Vegas there was little change—until you started gambling at the crap table. Then your heart rate jumped to 180 per minute and remained that way during the entire time you were gambling. It only dipped when you were escorted from the table and tried to explain yourself to the management. Fortunately, there's absolutely no evidence of ischemia or strain on your heart. So, judging from *this* EKG stress test, you have excellent cardiac function without any evidence of coronary insufficiency. Whether you're gambling at the crap table or, presumably, gambling in the stock market, these palpitations are, at the present time, perfectly harmless, and your heart tolerates them beautifully."

"O.K.," Blake said. "This EKG stress test I'll believe."

In spite of the extreme tension of his profession, he did not strike me as a Type A personality. He was more like a performer who does a high-wire act. Once he's done his act for the day, it's forgotten until the next day, and he then relaxes totally.

Blake insisted on taking me to lunch. It was not simply a token of gratitude from a patient. Not with Christopher Blake. He wanted to hear more about the newer devices and concepts in cardiology, and he figured that if he could nail me to a chair for an hour—he was prepared to buy me the best lunch in town—he might hear more about things that had caught his imagination. It was another con, but one I enjoyed.

He was amazed when I told him about the effects of the mind on the body and the new biofeedback devices just beginning to be used to control angina pectoris and hypertension. By attaching patients to devices where, for example, their heart rate could be continuously recorded and played back to them simultaneously, they could be trained to either slow or speed up their heart rate.

"My God," he exclaimed. "Isn't that what the yogis do?"

"Exactly," I responded. "We steal from anybody." I smiled. "Biofeedback is still in its scientific infancy, but it may have monumental uses." I went on. "We may want to train people to control their brain waves and prevent some forms of epilepsy, or to control their heart rates so as to prevent anxiety or sudden fright from increasing the rate to dangerous levels."

"You know something, Harold," Blake said wonderingly, "all this stuff you've been telling me about heart gadgets, all this biofeedback stuff, makes you think of science fiction, doesn't it?"

"Yes, but it also makes me think of Aristole, a man who's been dead well over two thousand years."

"The Greek philosopher?"

"And the greatest scientific authority of the ancient world. He believed the heart was the seat of intelligence. When I was in medical school I thought that was pretty funny. But now when I see how subtly the heart forces us to alter our ways of thinking and behaving since we all want to keep our hearts healthy, I'm beginning to wonder if maybe he wasn't on to something."

Appendix I.
Sexual Activity

Q. Could the excitement of sex bring on another heart attack?

A. The chances are one in a million. Sexual activity is like any other form of exercise. If you gradually build your exercise tolerance, the stress placed upon the heart by sex becomes less and less. Your heart should have absolutely no problems in responding to the physical demands imposed by sexual activity if you increase the vigor of those activities gradually.

Q. Are there any specific symptoms that might happen during sexual activity that I should call to my physician's attention?

A. Certainly any unusual symptoms—such as sustained heart palpitations, undue breathlessness, chest pain—

that occur before, during, or after sexual activities. These symptoms are usually easily preventable or treatable and in no way should interfere with total readjustment to a normal happy and healthy sexual life.

Q. How soon after the heart attack can I return to my *usual* sexual activity?

A. Sex in one form or another can usually be initiated six to ten weeks after a heart attack. After a gradual buildup, your usual sexual activity level can generally be reached twelve to fourteen weeks following the heart attack.

Q. You mean I shouldn't start right away with full intercourse?

A. A gradual buildup is the wisest course. The technique requiring the least expenditure of physical effort is masturbation or mouth-genital contact. People who have personal objections to masturbation and oral sex should start with other more generally accepted forms of sexual activity, since tension and anxiety should, even in a negative way, not be generated at this juncture.

Q. Do heart attacks effect potency in the male?

A. Absolutely not. From a physiological point of view, a heart attack has absolutely no effect upon one's ability to perform adequately or to obtain full gratification from sexual activity. Sexual performance may be affected by the anxiety and apprehension that may accompany one's concern about his ability to perform adequately. If a man is anxious about resuming sexual activity, it may be difficult for him to have an erection. But this is not a physical problem, and it will usually disappear with time.

Q. Are there any special positions that are preferable?

A. For the first several weeks after beginning sexual activity, you should not try to support any significant weight, since that requires considerable effort. One way to avoid this is to have your sex partner take the dominant position. Lie on your back with your partner on top. By supporting herself or himself on forearms and knees your partner must keep most of the weight off you and play the active role. You can be concentrating on your breathing.

Q. Why do I have to concentrate on my breathing?

A. Strange as it seems, you should learn how to breathe properly before initiating sexual activity. You should try to consciously control the degree of panting, grunting, and respiratory maneuvers that usually accompany sexual activity so as not to increase the intrathoracic pressure, the pressure within your chest, which in turn may increase your heart rate or blood pressure. You should therefore practice mouth breathing, breathing slowly through your mouth and not through your nose.

Q. What difference does that make?

A. When you breathe through your mouth, you are unable to close your glottis, the small membrane in the back throat. We commonly close the glottis when straining—for example, when having a bowel movement or when we hold our breath when lifting objects. Intrathoracic pressure can be increased only if the glottis is closed, and this is exactly what the cardiac patient should avoid. It is therefore wise to learn to breathe slowly through the mouth when you are having sex.

Q. Are there special breathing techniques during orgasm?

A. It is *especially* important that at the time of climax you breathe slowly and deeply through your mouth. Let the physical effects of the orgasm occur from the waist down. Actually, many patients say that once they learn this they find it infinitely more gratifying than the orgasms they used to experience, and they frequently remark that it is followed by a sensation of total relaxation.

Q. Are there many positions that the cardiac can adopt?
A. Yes, there are several for the male. In one, the woman straddles the man, her legs are spread on either side of his legs and are doubled underneath. Thus, as she accepts his penetration she is not only giving herself strong additional support with her knees to prevent her weight from pressing down on him but she can readily assume a sitting position without disturbing their connection. In a second method, the woman sits above, with her legs spread and knees bent; but instead of facing him, she faces the same direction he does, so that during intercourse she is presenting him with her back. In a third method, the man sits in a chair that is low enough so that when the woman sits on his lap, either facing him or facing away, her feet are planted solidly on the floor. By bracing her legs, she can keep much of her weight off him. Another maneuver is for the couple to lie on their sides, face to face, side by side, with legs interlocked. The woman may put her upper leg over both the man's legs or she may put her lower leg between his legs. In a fifth maneuver, the woman lies on her side, her back to the man, presenting her buttocks to him, and pulls her knees up toward her chest. The man is then able to penetrate deeply from the rear with minimal effort.

Q. Is there anything I should tell my spouse that will put him or her at ease?

A. You can say that virtually all heart victims eventually return to their normal sexual activities without significant problems. In fact, many couples will learn new approaches to achieving sexual gratification which they ordinarily would not have considered before the heart attack. A heart attack can therefore herald the beginning of a second life for sexual activity, too.

Appendix II. Diet

Q. I know I'm going to have to change my eating habits because of my heart condition. It's not going to be much fun, is it?

A. Actually, if you put in any effort at all, you'll find your new way of eating can be much more interesting and fun. Thousands of controlled fat, low-cholesterol recipes are available. For example, *The American Heart Association Cookbook* (David McKay Co.) offers over 400 unusual recipes designed to lower saturated fats and cholesterol in the diet.

Q. Will I have to diet for the rest of my life?

A. "Diet" isn't the right word. "Changing your eating habits" is more correct and it needn't be an ordeal. You might have to eliminate excessive quantities of some foods, such as milk and eggs. But this is only changing *your way* of eating; you need no eliminate all the good things you like. You'll find that, after altering your diet and sticking to it for several months, you will not feel restricted or deprived. In fact, you'll probably be amazed at the variety of foods and recipes that are allowed and that you can comfortably consume without feeling guilty.

Q. Do I have to give up meat and eggs?

A. What you have to give up are saturated fats—fats that harden at room temperature and that tend to raise the level of cholesterol in the blood. Americans consume 40 to 45 percent of their calories every day in fats, most of them saturated. Saturated fats are found in most animal products such as beef, lamb, pork, ham, butter, cream, whole milk, and cheeses made from cream or whole milk. They are also found in some vegetable products, such as solid and hydrogenated shortenings, coconut oil, cocoa butter, and palm oil (which, incidentally, is used commercially in preparing cookies, pie fillings, and non-dairy milk or cream substitutes). The proper fat-controlled, low-cholesterol diet will have less fat and contain only 30 to 35 percent of the day's calories. So, the answer is, yes, you should cut way down on meat except fish, poultry, and veal, and you should limit yourself to three eggs a week and more of the fats in your diet should be polyunsaturated.

Q. What are polyunsaturated fats?

A. Polyunsaturated fats are usually found in liquid vegetable oils such as corn, cotton seed, safflower, sesame seed, soya bean, and sunflower seeds. A higher proportion of the fat you consume should be polyunsaturated, since they tend to lower the level of cholesterol in the blood.

Q. What foods should 1 avoid totally?

A. All foods that contain too much fat, the wrong kind of fat, or too much cholesterol. The following is a list of "avoids."

FOODS TO AVOID

These are the foods that are not allowed on your diet—because they contain too much fat, the wrong kind of fat, or too much cholesterol.

DO NOT USE

MEATS

Beef high in fat or "marbled"
Lamb high in fat
Pork high in fat
Bacon, salt pork, spareribs

Frankfurters, sausage, cold cuts
Canned meats
Organ meats such as kidney, brain, sweetbread, liver
Any visible fat from meat

POULTRY AND FISH

Skin of chicken or turkey
Duck and goose
Fish roe (including caviar)

Fish canned in olive oil

DAIRY FOODS

Whole milk, homogenized milk, canned milk
Sweet cream, powdered cream
Ice cream unless homemade with nonfat dry milk powder

Sour cream
Whole milk buttermilk and whole milk yogurt
Butter
Cheese made from whole milk

FATS AND OILS

Butter
Ordinary margarines
Ordinary solid shortenings
Lard

Salt pork
Chicken fat
Coconut oil
Olive oil
Chocolate

BREADS AND BAKERY GOODS

Commercial biscuits, muffins,
cornbreads, griddlecakes, waffles,
cookies, crackers
Mixes for biscuits, muffins,
and cakes (except angel food)

Coffee cakes, cakes (except angel
food), pies, sweet rolls,
doughnuts, and pastries

DESSERTS

Puddings, custards, and
ice creams unless homemade
with skim milk or nonfat
dry milk powder

Whipped cream desserts
Cookies unless homemade with
allowed fat or oil

MISCELLANEOUS

Sauces and gravies unless made
with allowed fat or oil or
made from skimmed stock
Commercially fried foods such
as potato chips, French
fried potatoes, fried fish
Cream soups and other
creamed dishes
Frozen or packaged dinners
Olives
Macadamia nuts
Avocado

Chocolate
Candies made with chocolate,
butter, cream, or coconut
Coconut
Foods made with egg yolk unless
counted as part of your
allowance
Fudge, chocolate
Commercial popcorn
Substitutes for coffee cream
(usually contain saturated fats
or hydrogenated vegetable oils)

Q. What kinds of food can I eat to my heart's content?

A. Since all foods contain calories and calories mean weight, you can eat to your "heart's content" only if you keep your weight normal. However, if you do maintain your proper weight, you should be able to eat virtually unlimited quantities of fish, poultry, or veal. You may eat all the vegetables and fruits you care to, fruit juices or cups, clear soups and vegetable salad oils. Get in the habit of saying no to fried foods, casseroles and other mixed dishes, creamed foods, cream soups, gravies, cheeses, ice cream, pudding, cake, pie, and similar desserts.

Q. Do I have to give up coffee and tea? alcohol?

A. Coffee and tea are cardiac stimulants, but they can be consumed in moderation. Alcohol tends to be a general depressant, but there is no reason why you cannot have a cocktail or two or some wine.

Q. Should I have to take any special vitamins or minerals?

A. No. Recently there has been a tendency for people to take Vitamin E. However, this has not been scientifically proven to be of any value in patients with cardiac disease.

Q. Can I take diet pills?

A. No! Diet pills should be strictly avoided. First of all, they are cardiac stimulants and, secondly, they have been demonstrated to be totally ineffective for most people.

Q. Will my family have to change their diet to accommodate me?

A. Not necessarily. However, following a fat-controlled, low-cholesterol diet will certainly do them no harm, and indeed they will probably find the diet diverse and interesting.

Q. I eat lunch out a lot. Are there proper ways of having my food cooked?

A. Yes, your main course should be boiled, broiled, or baked. You should avoid fried foods, casseroles, and other mixed dishes, cream foods, and gravies. For the first course, have clear soup, tomato juice, or a fruit cup. For dessert have fruit, sherbert, gelatin, or unfrosted angel food cake.

Q. What if I feel desperate and cheat?

A. Following your new diet need not be a difficult chore in any way. For instance, several major food companies have prepared frozen and packaged foods specifically for patients on a fat-controlled, low-cholesterol diet. In most circumstances, a physician will not object to a patient's "temporary insanity"—that is, to having an occasional corned beef sandwich or Quiche Lorraine. What I might call "judicious dietary neglect" is O.K. on occasion if it helps you produce an emotional feeling of well-being and to achieve the end result of reducing your serum cholesterol and maintaining your ideal weight.

Appendix III. Exercise

Q. Is exercise dangerous for a cardiac patient?

A. Exercise can be dangerous to some people, but only to a few. Research has shown that a proper exercise training program will significantly *decrease* the chances of an individual sustaining a second heart attack. As a rule, the cardiac patient who has trained himself to the point of cardiovascular fitness will feel better and sleep better, and his outlook on life seems to improve. Certainly, before starting an exercise program, you should have a complete checkup, especially of the cardiovascular system. Like small plane flying, most of the problems occur not because of the activity but because of the performer. Joint pains, muscle aches, charley-horses and other things resulting from trying to do too much won't hurt you. However, one significant cardiac episode could *forever* dampen the enthusiasm of even the most fervent exercise freak.

Q. How much exercise can my heart take?

A. It varies from person to person. We want to produce cardiovascular fitness, but we also want to avoid exercise that is overly strenuous. It's dangerous to push yourself beyond exhaustion and fatigue, to the point where the heart and circulation can't deliver any more oxygen to the tissues—that point is known as the point of maximal aerobic power. That's when the lungs are putting oxygen into the bloodstream, but the blood can't transport the oxygen to the muscles fast enough to create energy for exercise. The muscles simply cannot receive any more oxygen then they are already getting. At about the same time that the oxygen supply becomes limited, the heart becomes essentially unable to beat any faster. That rate is called the maximal attainable heart rate—and *that* is certainly what you don't want to exceed.

Q. How do I know how much exercise to do?

A. Everyone has a target zone where he or she performs enough activity to achieve fitness, to condition the muscles and cardiovascular system, but that is not too vigorous to exceed safe limits. The target zone is considered between 70 and 85 percent of the maximal attainable heart rate.

Q. How do I determine my target zone?

A. First calculate your maximal attainable heart rate. A rough way to do this is to subtract your age from 220. For a fifty-year-old man, the maximal attainable heart rate is therefore 170 heartbeats per minute

(220 – 50 = 170). Thus, the 70 percent level is 119 heartbeats per minute and the 85 percent level is 145 heartbeats per minute. A fifty-year-old man, then, should program his exercise to bring his heart rate to between 119 and 145 beats per minute. An older person may expend the same degree of effort, but the heart rate will be considerably less.

Q. What's the best way to determine my heart rate?

A. Heart rates can be counted by simply taking your pulse for ten seconds and multiplying the result by six to get the heartbeats per minute. You should count the pulse *immediately* upon stopping your exercise because the heart rate changes very quickly once exercise is stopped.

Q. Where is the best place to take my pulse?

A. The pulse may be taken in any one of several places—on the thumb side of the wrist, on the side of the neck (place either thumb on your chin and feel the carotid artery in front of the muscle running vertically on both sides of the neck), inside the bend of the elbow, or in the groin. The count will always be the same no matter where you are counting.

Q. Once I determine my target zone, what next?

A. To achieve cardiovascular fitness, it is crucial that you exercise within the target zone for twenty to thirty minutes each session. First warm up slowly for five to ten minutes. This prevents undue stress on the heart and circulation, as well as soreness in the muscles and joints. Then step up the exercise, shooting for 70 to 75 percent of the maximal heart rate and maintain it there twenty minutes. Then gradually lessen the intensity of the exercise for the last five to ten minutes before stopping. This cool-down period will prevent minor but occasionally frightening symptoms such as dizziness, lightheadedness, nausea, all of which may occur if exercise is discontinued too abruptly.

Q. How do I actually start exercising?
A. Start a pattern that is easy and that doesn't fatigue you. The specific steps are as follows: Perform that exercise for five to ten minutes, then immediately take your pulse. The pulse rate should be less than 50 percent of your maximal attainable heart rate. Then exercise more vigorously for three to five minutes and take your pulse again. This time the pulse should be less than 70 percent of your maximal attainable heart rate. Again, exercise more strenuously for three to five minutes. If this time it is *above* 85 percent of your maximum, exercise more slowly or less vigorously. For example, reduce your running to a jog, or your jog to a brisk walk. In other words, upgrade or downgrade your exercise until you find out how much exercise is necessary to put you in the target zone, 70 to 85 percent of the maximal attainable heart rate. It may take several weeks to learn exactly how much effort it takes to get you to your target zone. You should continue to count the pulse rate religiously.

Q. What kind of exercises should I do?
A. Anything that is dynamic, that can be sustained, and that is aerobic. Dynamic exercises are always rhythmic and repetitive and, unlike static or isometric exercises, they involve motion. The exercise should be one that can be performed for relatively prolonged periods of time and it should be aerobic—that is, adequate oxygen can be supplied to the exercising muscles for as long as the exercise is performed. An activity is aerobic if it can

be continued for more than two or three minutes without significant shortness of breath or fatigue—for instance, jogging, bicycle riding, and swimming. Sprinting or rapid swimming from a cold start are not aerobic exercises since they cannot be performed at that pace for very long.

Q. Can I confine my exercises to weekends?

A. Absolutely not. Exercise should be carried out at least three times a week with no more than two days between workouts. At thirty minutes per day, that comes to at least ninety minutes per week.

Q. Is there any time when I should or shouldn't exercise?

A. You must *not* exercise for at least one hour after eating. That's an absolute cardinal rule. Thus, most people find the best time to exercise is before breakfast or before supper.

Q. How long will it take me to develop "perfect" cardiovascular fitness?

A. About three to six months, with a dedicated exercise program. But after only two to three weeks your level of physical fitness will improve. And after four to six weeks, you'll find that you're able to carry out the exercise more easily and that more exercise is required for you to reach your target zone. Many people say they are able to sleep better, are less fatigued during the day, and miss the invigorating feeling that comes from a good workout if they skip exercise for more than one or two days.

Q. Will I always do the same exercise?

A. As training progresses, the intensity of the exercise must be increased or your progress will come to a screeching halt. You may have to run instead of jog, swim more vigorously, and so on, in order to achieve the target zone. Any activity that achieves the target zone for twenty minutes or so is appropriate, but you have to train for it. Thus, changing exercises—for instance, substituting a rowing machine for jogging—may mean periods of retraining.

Q. Exercise bores me. How long will I have to continue it?

A. A cardiac patient usually has motivation enough because he wants to avoid a second coronary. However, whether you are cardiac or noncardiac, you should, of course, take up exercise you find enjoyable. Bicycling, tennis, swimming, jogging can all be fun if you do it with people you enjoy. Even with nonrecreational exercises, the boredom can be alleviated; for example, while you're riding a stationary bicycle you can watch television. Many people use their daily activities for exercise. One famous cardiologist, for example, never used elevators; he would climb the ten flights to his office twice daily at a pretty fast clip. Since this type of exercise is not sustained, however, he also supplemented the stair-climbing with fifteen-minute brisk walks three times a week.

Q. I love competitive athletics. Do I have to give them up?

A. Not necessarily. It depends on the demands placed on the heart by the particular sport. Most cardiac patients are able to get back to competitive sports such as tennis, baseball, and golf. However, downhill skiing may be intermittently extremely stressful and competitive handball, squash, hockey or basketball are usually highly stressful; few people are able to return to these sports without some risk. Still, some persons achieve a state of

cardiovascular fitness that will enable them to participate in all sports, even those of a highly competative
nature.

Q. Which sports are best for me to pursue now?

A. When you first start your program of conditioning, the
best "sport" is card playing but you should rapidly be
able to return to activities such as bowling, golfing,
horseback riding, bicycling, sailing, badminton, table
tennis, doubles court tennis, and canoeing.

Q. O.K., let's look at exercise. What's the best way to run
or jog?

A. Pick a flat street near you and measure off a mile, using
your car odometer. Then walk (don't run) that mile
continuously at the most rapid pace at which you are
comfortable. If it takes an hour, you're walking a rate of
one mile per hour. If you have not reached your target
zone, gradually increase the mile walk to twenty
minutes, which is three miles per hour. You might then
walk two miles in forty minutes, which is still three
miles an hour. After that, increase the rate to four or
even five miles per hour, which is a jog. Remember, the
target zone is always your endpoint.

Q. What about swimming or bathing?

A. Swimming, yes. Bathing, no. Bathing is simply paddling
or floating. Swimming is an excellent conditioning
activity, although it is dependent on your efficiency
(coordination and smoothness) and speed. Start by picking any stroke you're comfortable with, swim for five to
ten minutes, and then check your heart rate. After this
warm-up, you may swim more vigorously. After a few
sessions, you'll be able to swim for the entire twenty- to

thirty-minute period of exercise after your warm-up. Be sure to stay in the water for at least five to ten minutes after your swimming in order to "cool down."

Q. How about an indoor stationary bicycle?

A. Bicycling is superb exercise, but adjusting the device is important. Be sure the seat height and handlebar position are correct, so that you can concentrate on the exercise and not be bothered by discomfort. You'll know the seat height is correct when there is a small bend in your knee when your toe is on the down pedal. When the handlebar is positioned properly the body should be relaxed and slightly leaning forward. Always set the resistence knobs or dials at the lowest level for your warm-up until you have become conditioned to start at higher levels. Take your pulse rate after three or four minutes at each level and then increase the resistence level until you're able to achieve your target zone heart rate. Avoid electric bicycles that turn the peddles for you; they have nothing to offer you or your heart.

Q. How do I bicycle outdoors?

A. Follow the same rules as for indoors. Remember, however, that the exercise depends on the intensity of your peddling and whether you're going up and down hills. Thus, plan your route so that you can be on a flat stretch for five or ten minutes during your warm-up, then up and down hill for the next fifteen or twenty minutes, then back to a flat area for the end.

Q. I heard that skipping rope is a good exercise.

A. Ten minutes of vigorous rope skipping may be equivalent to thirty minutes of jogging, in relationship to cardiovascular fitness. The rope should be long enough so that when you stand on it, it reaches under the armpits. The basic jump is just high enough for the rope to pass under the feet and may be only an inch off the floor, but there are a variety of foot skills or jumping patterns. Warm up by jumping in place without the rope for 100 times. Then skip rope fifty times at a comfortable speed, increasing the number of skips ten per day so that at the end of five days, you will have reached ninety skips. Then reduce your warm-up to only fifty hops, and then do 100 skips per day, adding ten per day over the next five days until you have reached 140 per day. You may then enter an exercise period where after a warm-up of fifty hops, you skip 100 times, rest fifteen to thirty seconds, and then repeat 100 skips. Following five or six days of this routine, you may continue to add skips to the point of breathlessness, with an ultimate aim of reaching 500 skips in five minutes.

Q. Should I take frequent rests while I'm playing sports?

A. It depends on the sport. Some sports are extraordinarily demanding. You'll be able to determine this by taking your pulse rate and making certain that you're not above 85 percent of your maximal attainable heart rate. If you reach this level or exceed it, you'll obviously have to pull back by resting. If you do not reach the 70 percent level, there is no need to take frequent rests. Obviously, you should not play long enough to exhaust yourself, even though you may not reach the upper limits of the target zone. You may require more frequent rest when you first start playing the particular sport.

Q. What are the relative values of various exercises?

A. It is simple to calculate the value of certain exercises comparing them to the resting energy costs of simply lying in bed. We term these values *Mets,* which simply means the multiples of resting energy requirements. For example, an exercise that is in the energy range of three Mets will require three times the resting energy cost. However, these are relative average values only. The table shows the energy values for the various kinds of activity.

ACTIVITY

Energy range: 1.5-2 Mets. Usually not strenuous enough to produce endurance unless patient is elderly and capacity is very low. In addition, exercise is unsustained and ineffective in promoting endurance.

Occupational Activity	*Recreational Activity*
Desk work	Standing
Automobile driving	Strolling at 1 m.p.h.
Typing	Flying
Electric calculator machine operation	Motorcycling
	Playing cards
Light housework such as polishing furniture, sweeping, dusting	Sewing
	Knitting

Energy range: 2-3 Mets. These activities are usually intermittent and inadequately stressful to promote endurance, although they may promote muscular conditioning.

Occupational Activity	*Recreational Activity*
Auto repair	Level walking at 2 m.p.h.
Radio, TV repair	Level bicycling at 5 m.p.h.
Janitorial work	Riding lawnmower
Manual typing	Billiards
Bartending	Bowling
	Skeet

Shuffleboard
Woodworking, light
Power boat driving
Golf with a power cart
Canoeing at 2½ m.p.h.
Horseback riding
Bait casting
Playing a piano and other musical
   instruments

Energy range: 3-4 Mets. Walking and cycling at these levels is excellent dynamic exercise if the capacity is relatively low. Several of the other activities such as pushing a light power mower and housecleaning can be conditioning if carried out *continuously* for 20 to 30 minutes.

Occupational
Activity

Brick laying, plastering
Wheelbarrow, 100 lb. load
Machine assembly
Trailer-truck in traffic
Welding, moderate load
Cleaning windows

Recreational
Activity

Walking at 2½ m.p.h.
Cycling at 6 m.p.h.
Horseshoe pitching
Volleyball, six-man noncompetitive
Golf, pulling bag cart
Archery
Sailing, handling small boat
Fly fishing, standing with waders
Horseback, "sitting" to trot
Badminton, social doubles
Pushing light power mower
Energetic musician

Energy range: 4-5 Mets. Walking and cycling are, of course, excellent dynamic aerobic exercises. Calisthenics will promote endurance if continuous, rhythmic, and repetitive. However, exercises such as push-ups and sit-ups are probably not beneficial for cardiovascular fitness unless sustained and taxing from a cardiovascular point of view. Doubles tennis is of questionable benefit unless play is continuous and target cardiac rate is achieved.

Occupational
Activity

Painting, masonry
Paperhanging
Light carpentry

Recreational
Activity

Walking at 3 m.p.h.
Cycling at 8 m.p.h.
Table tennis

Golf, carrying clubs
Dancing, foxtrot
Badminton, singles
Tennis, doubles
Raking leaves
Hoeing
Many calisthenics

Energy range: 5-6 Mets. Properly performed walking, cycling, ice or roller skating, and yard work can be dynamic aerobic exercises if performed continuously for at least 20 to 30 minutes.

Occupational Activity	*Recreational Activity*
Digging garden	Walking at 3½ m.p.h.
Shoveling light earth	Cycling at 10 m.p.h.
	Canoeing at 3 m.p.h.
	Horseback, "posting" to trot
	Stream fishing, wading in light current in waders
	Ice or roller skating at 9 m.p.h.

Energy range: 6-7 Mets. Singles tennis can provide benefit if played 30 minutes or more by a skilled player with an attempt to keep moving. Water skiing is an isometric exercise and quite risky for a cardiac or a deconditioned normal. Snow shoveling should not be performed unless slowly smoothly, rhythmically, and a target heart rate zone should never be exceeded.

Occupational Activity	*Recreational Activity*
Shoveling 10 minutes, 10 lb.	Walking at 5 m.p.h.
	Cycling at 11 m.p.h.
	Badminton, competitive
	Tennis, singles
	Splitting wood
	Snow shoveling
	Hand lawn mowing
	Folk (square) dancing
	Light downhill skiing
	Ski touring, 2½ m.p.h. (loose snow)
	Water skiing

Energy range: 7-8 Mets. Ski runs for experienced skiers are usually too short to promote endurance. Combined stress of altitude, cold, and exercise may be too great for many cardiacs. Paddle tennis may be too stressful from a cardiac point of view because of competition and warm lights of playing area. However, if continuous, may be beneficial in reaching target heart rate.

Occupational Activity	*Recreational Activity*
Digging ditches	Jogging at 5 m.p.h.
Carrying 80 lb.	Cycling at 12 m.p.h.
Sawing hardwood	Horseback, gallop
	Vigorous downhill skiing
	Basketball
	Mountain climbing
	Ice hockey
	Canoeing at 4 m.p.h.
	Touch football
	Paddleball

Energy range: 8-9 Mets. Squash and handball may be too intermittent to provide endurance building effects and, competition associated with the warm lights in the playing area may be too stressful. Ski touring may also be too stressful for cardiacs since combined stress of altitude, cold and exercise may be excessive. Running and cycling continue to be excellent dynamic aerobic and endurance building exercises.

Occupational Activity	*Recreational Activity*
Shoveling 10 minutes, 14 lb.	Running at 5½ m.p.h.
	Cycling at 13 m.p.h.
	Ski touring, 4 m.p.h. (loose snow)
	Squash racquets, social
	Handball, social
	Fencing
	Basketball, vigorous

Energy range: 10+ Mets. Competitive handball and squash at these levels may be extremely dangerous to anyone who is not in excellent physical condition.

Occupational *Activity*	*Recreational* *Activity*
Shoveling 10 minutes, 16+ lb.	Running 6 m.p.h. = 10 Mets
	Running 7 m.p.h. = 11½ Mets
	Running 8 m.p.h. = 13½ Mets
	Running 9 m.p.h. = 15 Mets
	Running 10 m.p.h. = 17 Mets
	Ski touring, 5+ m.p.h. (loose snow)
	Handball, competitive
	Squash, competitive

Appendix IV.
Cigarette Smoking

Q. Why do I have to give up smoking?

A. Extensive research has suggested that smoking may accelerate the development of coronary atherosclerosis and also may trigger sudden death in persons with underlying coronary artery disease. For instance, between 1951 and 1965 about half the British doctors stopped smoking cigarettes, but most British males continued smoking. Among the doctors the death rate dropped 12.4 percent, whereas among the total male population of England, the death rate dropped only 3 percent. In addition, deaths from coronary heart disease declined 6 percent among the physicians but it increased 32 percent in the general male population.

Q. My grandmother smoked for over seventy years and she died when she was ninety-two, so I don't see why I would have any trouble.

A. She might have lived to be a hundred and ten. Every smoker is at a much higher risk of developing sudden death or other symptoms of coronary insufficiency. The risk of developing coronary heart disease is about 70 percent greater for smokers than for nonsmokers. And in men aged forty to forty-nine, smoking two packs of cigarettes a day increases the coronary heart disease mortality five times over that of the nonsmokers in the same age group.

Q. If you've been smoking for a long period of time, isn't it too late? Hasn't the damage already been done?

A. Your body has amazing recuperative abilities, and no matter how long or how much you've been smoking, your body will immediately begin the process of repair once you stop. Some damage may indeed already have occurred, but it certainly will not be as great as the damage that will occur if smoking is continued.

Q. What if I smoke only a small number of cigarettes per day? Is that O.K.?

A. Reducing your consumption to five cigarettes or less per day is probably helpful from a cardiac point of view. However, this is usually pretty difficult for a person who has smoked twenty to forty cigarettes a day. Most people will revert to their old habits.

Q. Does a filter make smoking safer?

A. In a minor way. Some filters remove the particulate matters in smoke and therefore may reduce the hazard of developing lung cancer. But many chemicals, particulate matter, and gases, such as carbon monoxide are not screened out by filters.

Q. Wouldn't it be just as good to switch to a low tar and nicotine cigarette?

A. It's possible that the reduction in the dose of these chemicals will reduce the associated risks of developing severe cardiopulmonary problems. But it is nowhere as good as simply discontinuing smoking totally. You might try a low tar and nicotine cigarette as a way of tapering off for two to four weeks before you stop entirely.

Q. What about switching to a pipe or cigar?

A. Pipes and cigars are rarely inhaled and so do not have the same risks as cigarettes. A pipe or cigar can be helpful in tiding you over the withdrawal from cigarettes. But if you inhale on it, you are no better off. Since pipe and cigar smokers have a higher risk of developing cancer of the mouth and oral cavity than do nonsmokers, I would recommend using a pipe or cigar only temporarily if at all.

Q. Isn't cigarette smoking somewhat addicting, like a drug?

A. Cigarette smokers are emotionally addicted to their habit but not physiologically addicted. Actually, they are "habituated." Your body does not demand cigarette smoke; thus, the ability to stop smoking depends upon having a significant motivation, an incentive to quit the habit.

Q. Whenever I stop smoking, I become extremely nervous. Why?

A. Smoking is a conditioned reflex. Over the years, you

learned to handle many tensions by smoking. You have to relearn how to handle these anxieties and not automatically reach for a cigarette.

Q. Are the physical symptoms I get when I quit smoking dangerous?

A. You mean shortness of breath, palpitations, vague chest pain, free-floating anxiety, headaches, lightheadedness, fatigue, sleeplessness, irritability? No, they're not dangerous, and after a week or two, they usually decrease dramatically. Many patients report immediate changes in their physical and emotional well-being as soon as they stop smoking. They note an immediate decrease in fatigue, insomnia, congestion in the upper respiratory passages, and in any chronic cough or hoarseness. Stamina seems to increase. Some patients even say that their face wrinkles improve or, at least, seem to develop more slowly.

Q. Should I stop smoking suddenly or taper off gradually?

A. Whatever works best for you.

Q. What about antismoking drugs? Will they help?

A. Stimulants, sedatives, and tranquilizers sometimes help the symptoms associated with smoking. Other drugs simulate the effects of nicotine or affect the taste sensations of smoking. There is no evidence that these tobacco substitutes make quitting easier, although some smokers say they help them over the withdrawal period. Many drugs require prescriptions and if taken in large doses or over prolonged periods of time are unsafe or addictive.

Q. Are there any good techniques to help me stop smoking?

A. Literally hundreds of so-called "sure fire" methods have developed over the years. There are books with self-training techniques—relearning processes that are self-taught—which are effective for some patients. There are smoking clinics which are structured teaching programs. Hypnosis has been used with variable success. Some commercial organizations have tried using aversion techniques such as an electric shock; these may be effective in the short term but not usually in the long run. The long-term results of these various methods have never been carefully studied from a scientific point of view. Certainly before you spend money on any of these techniques, you should try to see what you can do by yourself.

Q. If I stop smoking, I'll gain weight, won't I?

A. Not necessarily. In fact, some patients *lose* weight. If you have an especially deep need for oral gratification and find yourself overeating after you quit smoking, I would say "overeat"—*but only for a little while.* First, get rid of the smoking habit, then get rid of the over-eating habit. And, believe me, if you can stop smoking, you can control your eating.

Q. What if I fail and start smoking again?

A. It doesn't mean you'll be unable to stop permanently. Some people backslide several times before they finally stop once and for all.

Q. If I stop smoking, I might develop some other bad habit like alcoholism or drug addiction.

A. Baloney. If you can stop smoking you can do anything. Controlling the cigarette habit means you probably can control most other areas in your life.

Q. What the hell, we all have to die sometime. I enjoy smoking, and anyway I'm too old to give it up.

A. There's nothing we can do about dying, of course, but it seems stupid to die prematurely. Moreover, no one wants to die from a long, painful, illness.

Glossary

Angina pectoris: Condition in which the heart muscle receives an insufficient blood supply, causing pain in the chest and often in the left arm and shoulder.

Angiocardiography: X-ray examination of the heart and blood vessels which follows an opaque fluid injected into the bloodstream.

Aorta: Main trunk artery which receives blood from the lower left chamber of the heart.

Arteriosclerosis: "Hardening of the arteries." Includes a variety of conditions that cause the artery walls to thicken and lose elasticity.

Artery: Blood vessel that carries blood away from the heart to the various parts of the body.

Atherosclerosis: Form of arteriosclerosis. The inner layers of artery walls are made thick and irregular by fatty deposits. The internal channel of arteries becomes narrowed, and blood supply is reduced.

Atrium: Also called *auricle.* One of the two upper chambers of the heart.

Blood Pressure: Force exerted by the heart in pumping blood; the pressure of blood in the arteries.

Capillaries: Small blood vessels that distribute oxygenated blood to all parts of the body.

Cardiac: Pertaining to the heart.

Cardiac arrest: When heart stops beating; cessation of cardiac output and effective circulation.

Cardiopulmonary resuscitation: Combination of chest compression and mouth-to-mouth breathing. Used during fibrillation or cardiac arrest to keep oxygenated blood flowing to the brain until appropriate medical treatment can be initiated.

Cardiovascular: Pertaining to the heart and blood vessels.

Catheterization: The process of examining the heart by introducing a thin tube (catheter) into a vein or artery and passing it into the heart.

Cerebral thrombosis: Formation of a blood clot in a blood vessel leading to the brain.

Cholesterol: A fat-like substance found in animal tissue. In blood tests the normal level for Americans is between 180 and 230 milligrams per 100 cc. A higher level is often associated with a high risk of heart attack and stroke.

Cineangiography: The taking of movie pictures to show the passage of an opaque dye through blood vessels.

Circulatory system: Pertaining to the heart, blood vessels, and circulation of the blood.

Collateral circulation: System of smaller blood vessels which carry blood when a main blood vessel is blocked.

Congestive heart failure: Backing up of blood in the veins leading to the heart often accompanied by accumulation of fluid in various parts of the body. Results from the heart's inability to pump out all the blood that returns to it.

Coronary arteries: Two arteries, arising from the aorta, arching down over the top of the heart and conducting blood to the heart muscle.

Coronary care unit: In-hospital or emergency mobile unit, equipped with monitoring devices and staffed with trained personnel, designed to treat coronary patients.

Coronary occlusion: Obstruction or narrowing of one of the coronary arteries which hinders blood flow to some part of the heart muscle.

Coronary thrombosis: Also called *coronary occlusion.* Formation of a clot in one of the arteries that conduct blood to the heart muscle.

Cyanosis: Blueness of skin caused by insufficient oxygen in the blood.

Defibrillator: Agent or measure that stops an incoordinate contraction of the heart muscle and restablishes normal rhythm.

Diastolic pressure: Blood pressure level during time the heart muscle is relaxed.

Digitalis: Drug that strengthens contraction of the heart muscle, slows rate of contraction of the heart, and promotes the elimination of fluid from body tissues.

Diuretic: Drug that promotes the excretion of urine.

Edema: Swelling due to abnormally large amounts of fluid in the body tissues.

Electrocardiogram (EKG or ECG): A graphic record of electric impulses produced by the heart.

Embolus: Blood clot that forms in blood vessels in one part of the body and travels to another.

Fibrillation: Uncoordinated contractions of the heart muscle occurring when individual muscle fibers take up independent irregular contractions.

Heart attack: Coronary occlusion or obstruction (generally a blood clot) in one of the coronary arteries which reduces or stops the flow of blood to some area of the heart muscle (myocardium) and results in damage to or death of that area.

High blood pressure (hypertension): Unstable or persistent elevation of blood pressure above the normal range.

Hypertension (high blood pressure): Unstable or persistent elevation of blood pressure above normal range.

Myocardial infarction: Damaging or death of an area of the heart muscle (myocardium) resulting from a reduction in the blood supply reaching that area.

Myocardium: Muscular wall of the heart which contracts in order to pump blood out of the heart and then relaxes as the heart refills with returning blood.

Nitroglycerin: Drug that causes dilation of blood vessels, often used in the treatment of angina pectoris.

Occluded artery: One in which blood flow has been impaired by a blockage.

Open heart surgery: Surgery performed on the opened heart while the bloodstream is diverted through a heart-lung machine.

Pulmonary: Pertaining to the lungs.

Saturated fat: Fat not capable of absorbing additional hydrogen.

Sphygmomanometer: Instrument for measuring blood pressure.

Stethoscope: Instrument for listening to sounds within the body.

Systolic blood pressure: Pressure inside the arteries when the heart contracts at each beat.

Thrombosis: Formation or presence of a blood clot (thrombus) inside a blood vessel or cavity of the heart.

Thrombus: Blood clot that forms inside a blood vessel or cavity of the heart.

Vascular: Pertaining to the blood vessels.

Vein: Any one of a series of vessels of the vascular system which carries blood from various parts of the body back to the heart.

Ventricle: One of the two lower chambers of the heart.

Bibliography

Christian Bernard, M.D., *Heart Attack: You Don't Have to Die.* New York: Delacorte, 1972.

William A. Brams, M.D. *Managing Your Coronary.* Philadelphia: Lippincott, 1966.

Myron Brenton, *Sex and Your Heart.* New York: Coward-McCann, 1968.

Morris Fishbeing, M.D., *Heart Care.* Garden City, N.Y.: Hanover House, 1960.

Meyer Friedman, M.D., and Ray H. Rosenman, M.D., *Type A Behavior and Your Heart.* New York: Knopf, 1974.

Jess Lair, Ph.D., and Jacqueline Carey Lair, *Hey, God, What Should I Do Now?* Garden City, N.Y.: Doubleday, 1973.

Lawrence E. Lamb, M.D., *Your Heart and How to Live with It.* New York: Viking Press, 1969.

William Likoff, M.D., Bernard Segal, M.D., and Lawrence Galton, *Your Heart.* Philadelphia: Lippincott, 1972.

Hamilton Maule, *Running Scared.* New York: Saturday Review Press, 1972.

Walter McQuade and Ann Aikman, *Stress*. New York: Dutton, 1974.

Benjamin F. Miller, M.D., and Lawrence Galton, *Freedom from Heart Attack*. New York: Simon & Schuster, 1972.

Robert A. Miller, M.D., *How to Live with a Heart Attack (and How to Avoid One)*. Radnor, Pa.: Chilton, 1971.

Brendan Phibbs, M.D., *Human Heart: A Guide to Heart Disease*. St. Louis: C.V. Mosby, 1971.

Elmer Pinckney M.D., and Cathy Pinkney, *The Cholesterol Controversy*. Los Angeles: Sherbourne Press, 1973.

Jane Schoenberg and JoAnn Stichman, *How to Survive Your Husband's Heart Attack*. New York: David McKay, 1974.

Peter S. Steinorown, M.D., *Your Heart Is Stronger Than You Think*. New York: Cowles, 1970.

Everett Weiss, *Don't Worry About Your Heart*. New York: Random House, 1959.

Kester Yehuda, *Diary of a Heart Patient*. New York: McGraw-Hill, 1968.